Cystic Fibrosis - Facts, Management and Advances

Edited by Prashant Mohite, Anna Reed and André R. Simon

Published in London, United Kingdom

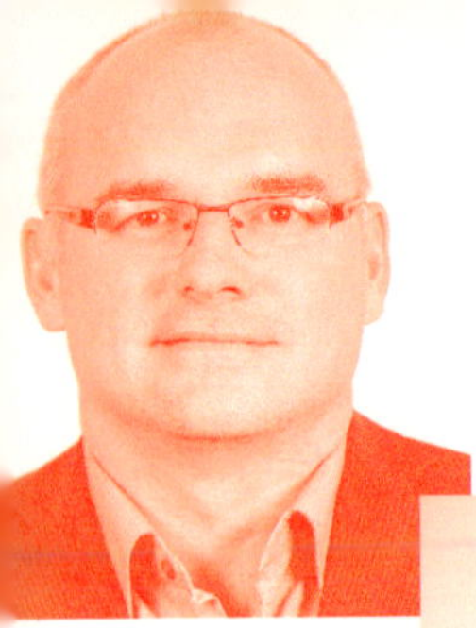
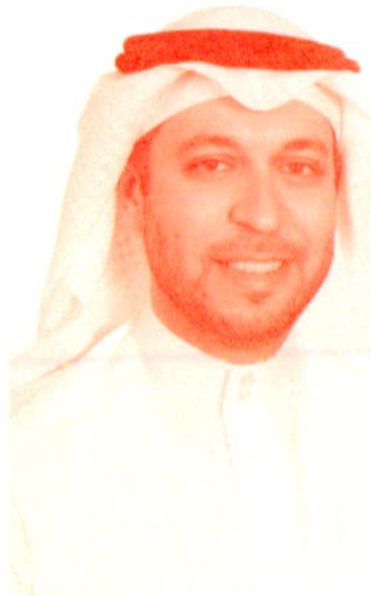
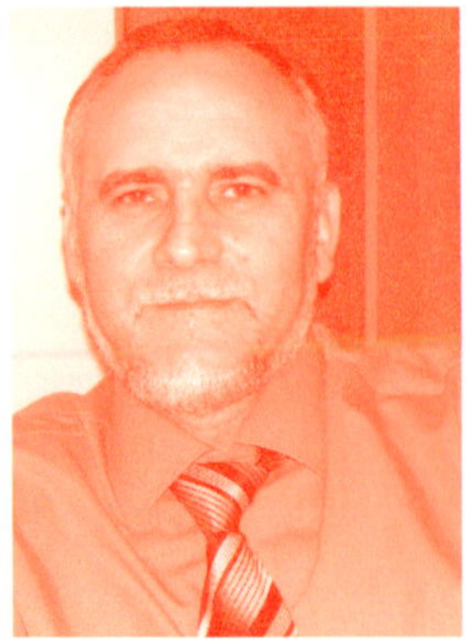
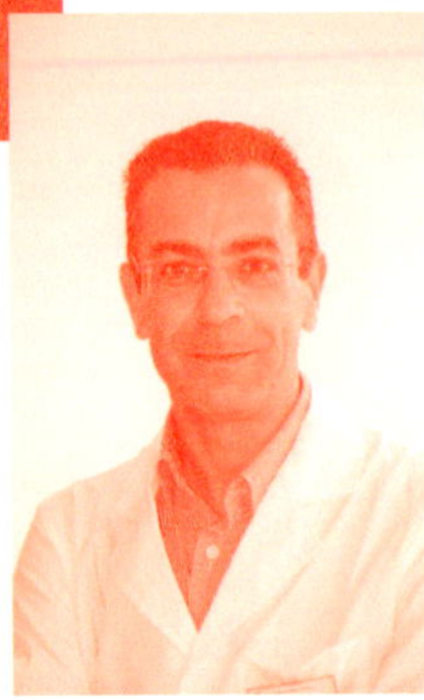
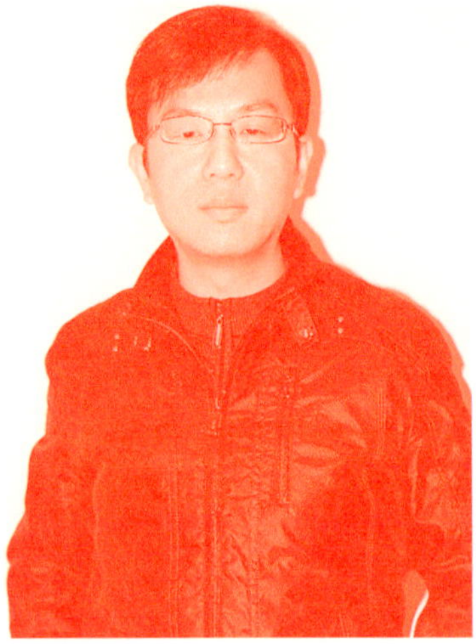
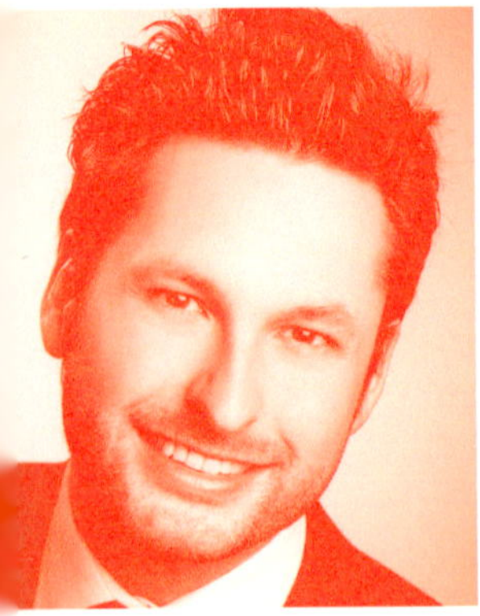
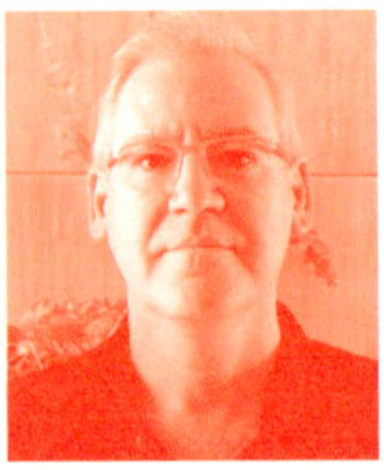

IntechOpen

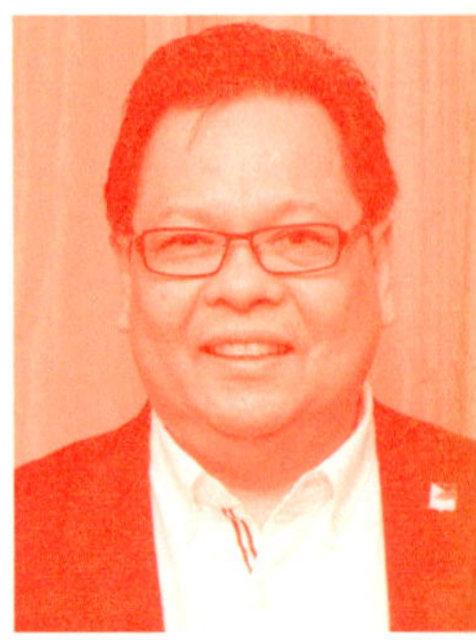
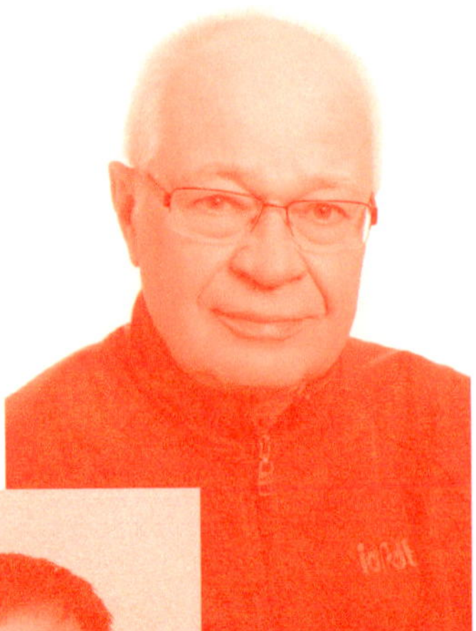
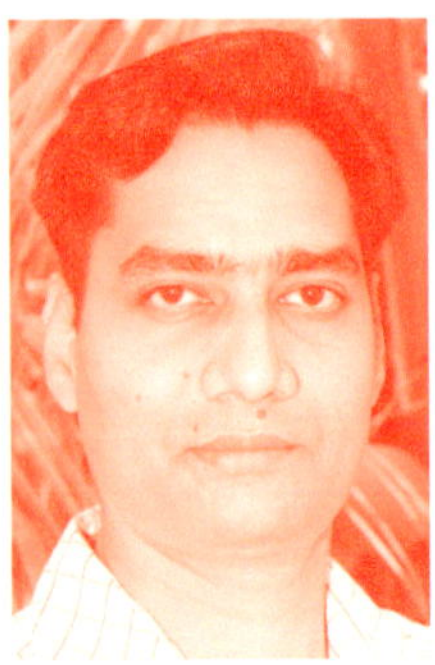
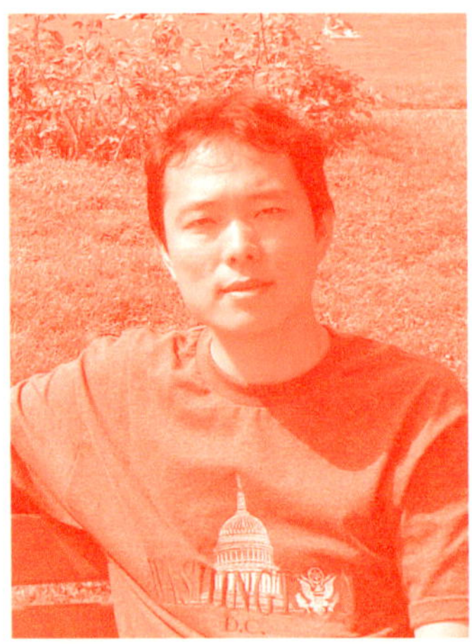
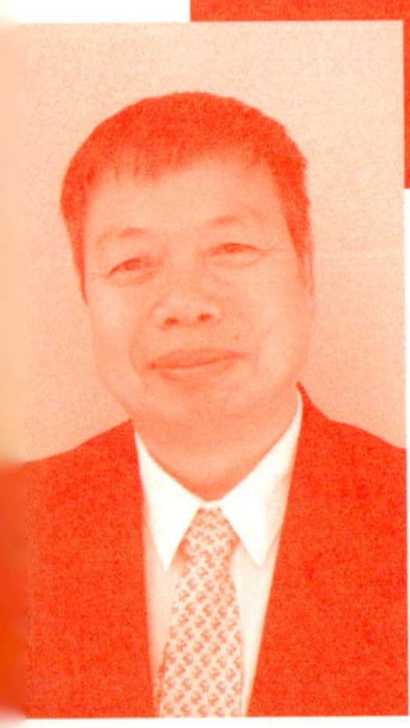
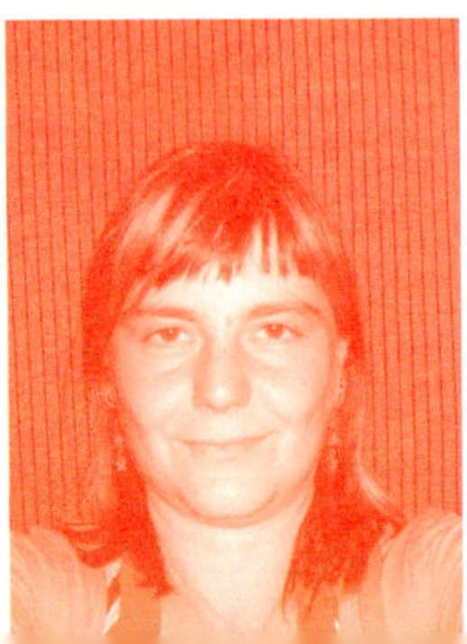

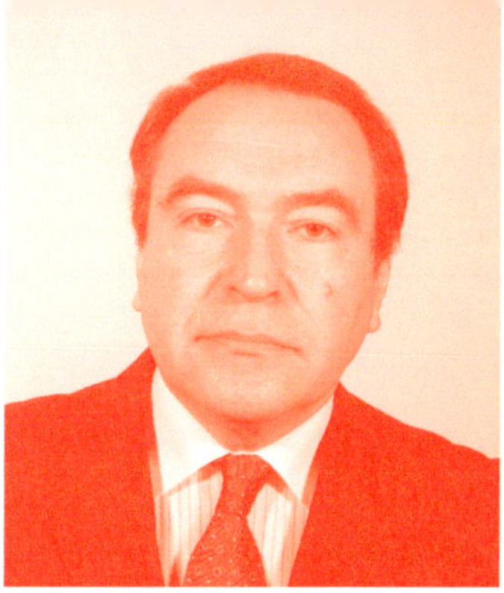
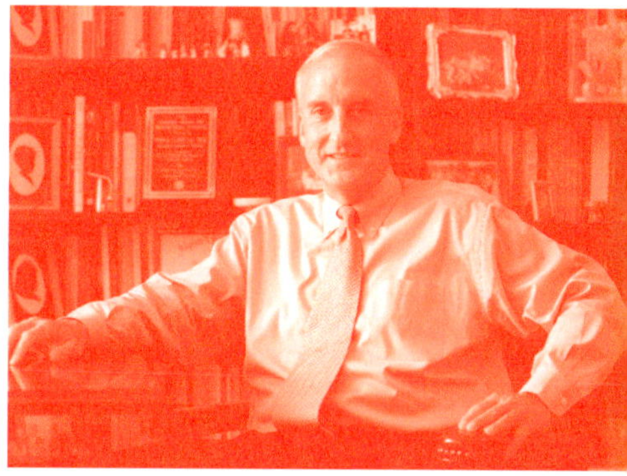
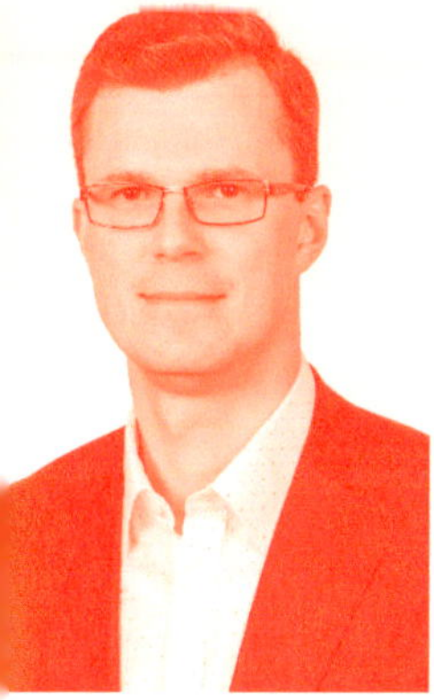
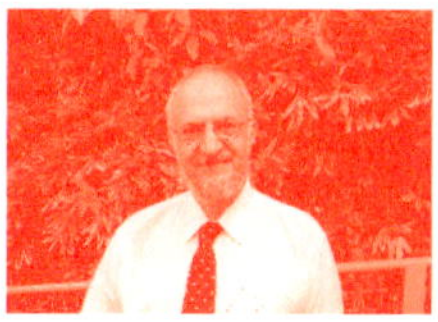
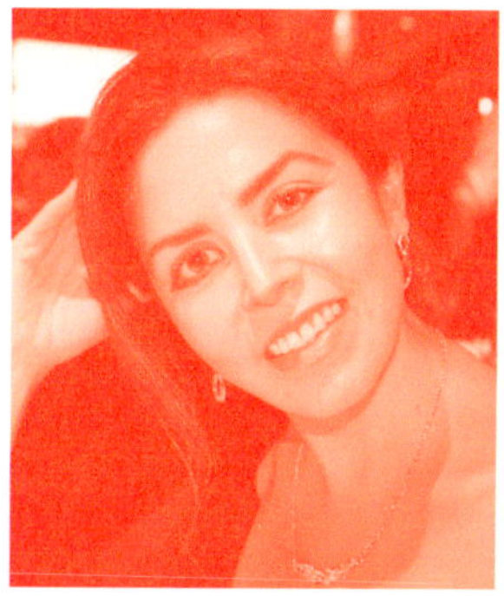

Supporting open minds since 2005

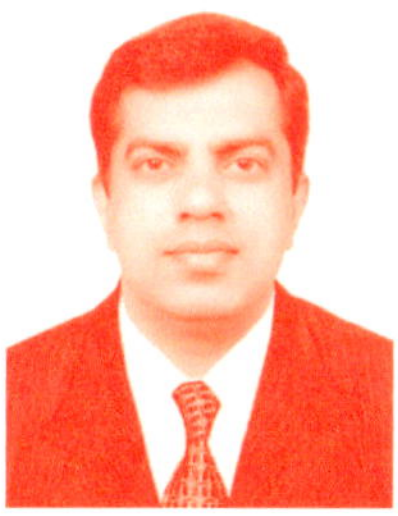
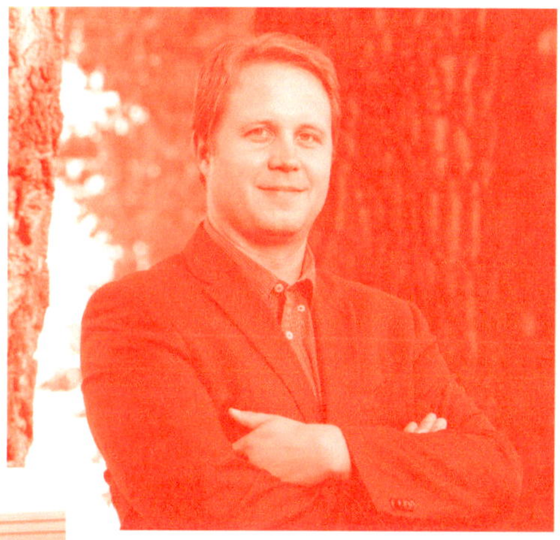
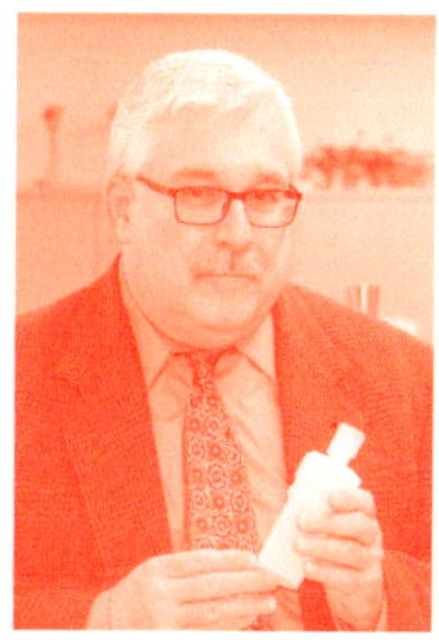
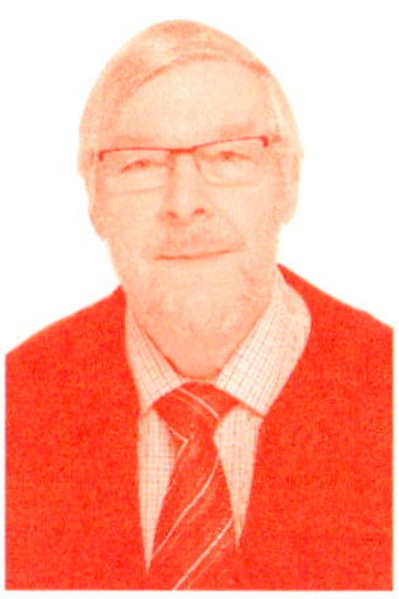
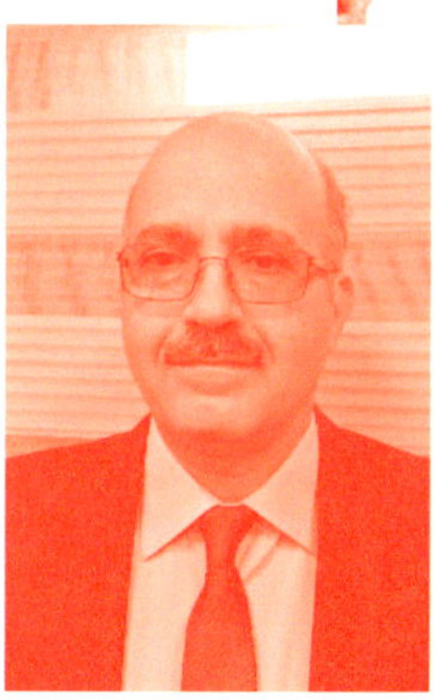
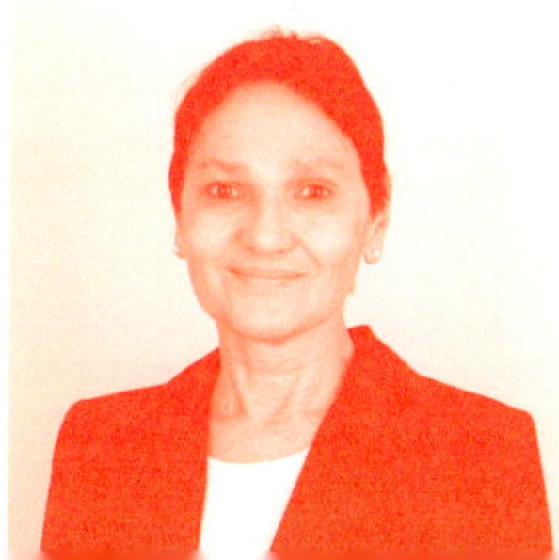
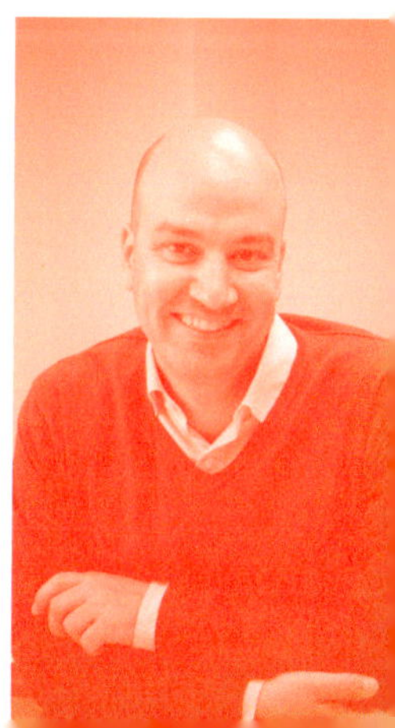

Cystic Fibrosis - Facts, Management and Advances
http://dx.doi.org/10.5772/intechopen.87623
Edited by Prashant Mohite, Anna Reed and André R. Simon

Contributors
Manfred Ballmann, Prashant N. Mohite, Anna Reed, André R. Simon, Kavita Dave, Waleed Mohamed Hussain Abdulkhair, Mousa Abdullah Alghuthaymi, Aris Tagalakis, Salsabil Elboraie, Konstantinos Kafetzis, Rajeev Shrivastava, Shihab Hameed, Katerina Theocharous, Bernadette Prentice, Charles F. Verge, Adam Jaffe, Vicky Gerovasili

First published in London, United Kingdom, 2021 by IntechOpen
IntechOpen is the global imprint of INTECHOPEN LIMITED, registered in England and Wales, registration number: 11086078, 5 Princes Gate Court, London, SW7 2QJ, United Kingdom
Printed in Croatia

British Library Cataloguing-in-Publication Data
A catalogue record for this book is available from the British Library

Additional hard and PDF copies can be obtained from orders@intechopen.com

Cystic Fibrosis - Facts, Management and Advances
Edited by Prashant Mohite, Anna Reed and André R. Simon
p. cm.
Print ISBN 978-1-83881-073-3
Online ISBN 978-1-83881-074-0
eBook (PDF) ISBN 978-1-83881-075-7

For EU product safety concerns:
IN TECH d.o.o., Prolaz Marije Krucifikse Kozulić 3, 51000 Rijeka, Croatia, info@intechopen.com or visit our website at intechopen.com.

Meet the editors

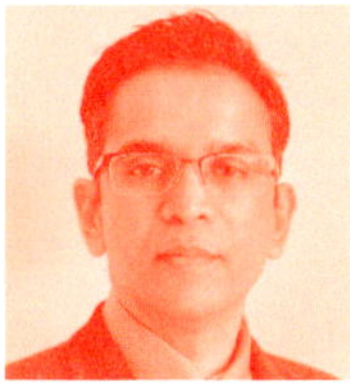

Prashant Mohite is trained as a cardiac surgeon in India and works as a Locum Consultant in Cardiac Retrieval at Golden Jubilee National Hospital. He was involved in the development of several programs at Harefield Hospital, England, including Organ Care Systems for heart and lungs, ex vivo lung perfusion, awake extracorporeal life support (ECLS), ECLS as a bridge to lung transplant, and donation after cardiac death (DCD) heart transplantation. He is an avid researcher having published in well-known journals and presented at multiple national and international meetings as an invited speaker as well as through voluntary abstract submissions.

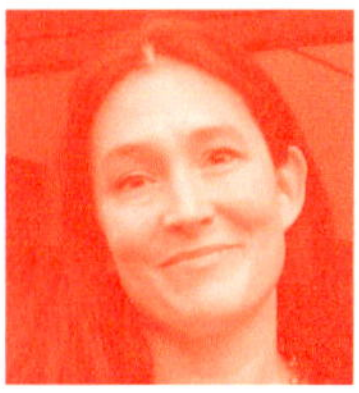

Dr. Anna Reed is a consultant in respiratory and transplant medicine, based at Harefield Hospital, England. She graduated from Leeds University in 1998 and obtained a Ph.D. in Pulmonary Vascular Pharmacology from Imperial College London in 2011. She maintains an active research interest in areas such as surfactant flux in primary graft dysfunction, ECMO bridging to lung transplant, pharmacokinetic and pharmacodynamic alterations of commonly used anti-infectives on extracorporeal life support, Aspergillus disease and the immunological impact on the transplanted lung, and more. She has authored multiple manuscripts in high-profile journals and has reviewed numerous journal articles.

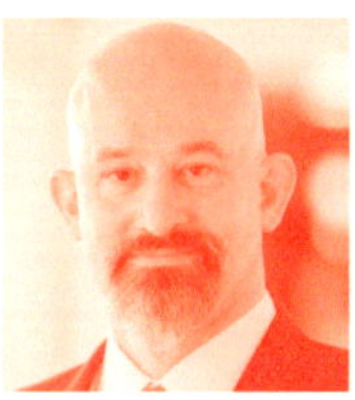

André R. Simon is a consultant cardiac surgeon and dircctor of heart and lung transplantation and ventricular assist devices at Harefield Hospital, England. He is also an honorary senior lecturer at Imperial College London. He has written more than 100 peer-reviewed papers, reviews, and editorials. He has also contributed chapters to several textbooks. He has raised more than £2 million in funding for research into transplantation immunology, cardiac imaging, and ventricular assist devices. Dr. Simon is the founder and president of HeartHelp, a charitable non-government organization.

Contents

Preface

Cystic fibrosis is a genetic disorder affecting multiple systems in the body with various levels of severity. Over the last few decades, the patterns of presentation, aspects of diagnosis, and approaches to its management have changed substantially. Rather than an acute disease in children, cystic fibrosis is also now a chronic condition in adults. In the developed world there are more adults than children affected with the disease. As more affected children are reaching adulthood, the burden on healthcare is ever increasing given the natural history of cystic fibrosis, which is riddled with exacerbations and complications requiring constant clinical input, healthcare professional visits, and frequent hospital admissions. The treatment of cystic fibrosis has also changed greatly over the years. Gene therapy that remained on the horizon for many years is now a reality in clinical practice. Current management is focused on preventing disease complications rather than treating them.

Today, the medical community is facing new challenges in the management of cystic fibrosis. The disease exhibits as a chronic affair with slow-deteriorating stable phases interspersed with acute exacerbations. These aspects of the disease mandate close observation and timely intervention at early signs of exacerbations to prevent catastrophic complications. Cystic fibrosis transforms the lungs into a hotbed for a variety of microbial flora that slowly develops resistance to multiple antibiotics. Advances in lung transplantation, immunosuppression, and post-operative management have led to increased survival rates for lung transplant recipients, qualifying more and more recipients as candidates for re-transplantation.

Since cystic fibrosis affects multiple bodily systems, its management naturally involves multiple specialties including genetics, microbiology, neonatology, pediatrics, diabetology, gastroenterology, infertility, psychiatry, respiratory, thoracic surgery, and transplant surgery. This volume serves as a handbook as well as a reference for clinicians, medical professionals, healthcare assistants and trainees in these various specialties. This covers the basics of the included as well as examines recent advances in the field. As "a picture is worth a thousand words," we have included in this book appropriate clinical photographs, explanatory cartoons, flowcharts, and diagrams. The book offers a comprehensive view of cystic fibrosis for students, professionals, and patients alike. We congratulate and thank all the authors who have contributed to this work.

Prashant Mohite, Anna Reed and André R. Simon
Royal Brompton and Harefield NHS Foundation Trust,
United Kingdom

Dedication

Dedicated to Smita, Christian, and Kirsten who sacrificed our company during the creation of this book.

-Prashant, Anna, and André

Chapter 1

Introductory Chapter: Basics of Cystic Fibrosis

Prashant N. Mohite and Vicky Gerovasili

1. Introduction

"Woe to the child who tastes salty from a kiss on the brow, for he is cursed and soon must die," describes European folklore and medical texts of middle ages a condition then unknown. It took several centuries for this condition to get its formal name from an American Pathologist Dr. Dorothy Anderson- cystic fibrosis [1]. While conducting an autopsy of a child apparently died of Celiac disease, she found '*cystic fibrosis of the pancreas*' and her later research for over a decade defined the characteristics of the disease that involved pancreas, lungs and intestine [2]. Dr. Paul di Sant'Agnese in 1948 New York heatwave noticed a higher concentration of salt in the sweat of dehydrated children leading to the first, most reliable and yet ubiquitously used 'sweat test' for the CF [3]. Dr. Anderson recognized that the disease is autosomal recessive, however, after half a century in 1989 Lap-Chee Tsui in Canada discovered a gene called CFTR (CF transmembrane conductance regulator), a mutation of which was responsible to cause CF [4]. Unfortunately, it was not the Holy Grail in the management of the CF as another 2000 variants of the gene mutation were found later on.

Even until the early part of the last century children affected with CF died of malnutrition. Discovery of pancreatic enzyme supplements and introduction of high-fat diet improved nutrition in CF children with many reaching to adulthood shifting the challenge to the pulmonary disease of CF. As more patients were diagnosed with the condition, a lot of organizations were founded in the western world to educate, support and treat CF. In 1965, the Royal Brompton hospital in London was the first in Europe, probably in the world to offer adult CF service [5]. Lack of knowledge and modern medicine in that era led to therapies like 'mist tent' where humidified air was delivered to liquefy mucus and 'upside-down postural drainage' to hasten expectorations. Over the decades, the discovery of various bugs affecting airways of CF patients and newer and more effective antibiotics to cull the bugs along with effective ways to deliver them including systematic inhalation saved many lives. The biggest breakthrough in the treatment of CF arrived at the beginning of the current century when gene therapy directed at fixing the defect in the gene was successfully implemented [6, 7]. Early detection and management with a well-organized nutrition plan, improved airway clearance, targeted, combination and tailored antibiotic therapy along with ever-developing gene therapy should significantly improve survival in the CF patients.

2. Pathophysiology of cystic fibrosis

In the past, CF was called as 'mucoviscidosis' and the term quite aptly underlines the pathophysiology of the disease. The CF is an autosomal recessive disorder that

IntechOpen

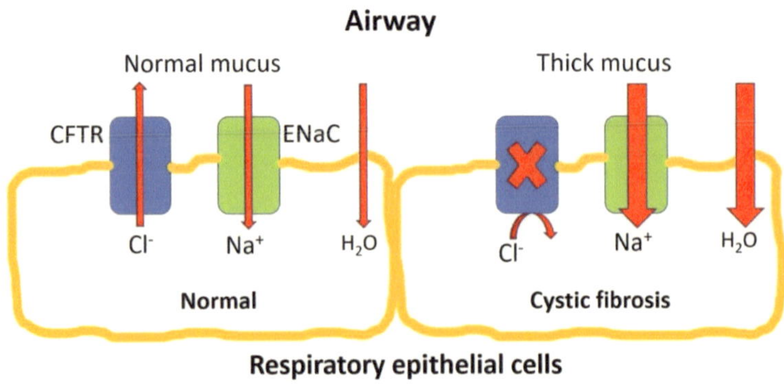

Figure 1.
Pathophysiology of cystic fibrosis.

transpires due to mutation in the CFTR gene on chromosome 7 [8]. The CFTR is an anion channel on the surface of the epithelial cells that regulate cyclic AMP-dependent and ATP energized secretion of chloride ions (Cl-) outside the cell and epithelial sodium channel (ENaC) regulated entry of Sodium ion (Na+) into the cell [9]. Simply put, the mutation in the gene leads to less secretion of chloride ion and inappropriate absorption of the sodium ion into the epithelial cells creating hyperosmolarity inside the cell and dehydration on its surface (**Figure 1**). F508del recognized by the absence of phenylalanine at position 508 in CFTR accounts for about two-thirds of mutations while the rest of the mutations measures less than 5% individually [10]. Manifestations of CF involving various systems in the body are due to this genetic defect causing epithelial surface dehydration related viscid mucus.

3. Clinical picture of cystic fibrosis

In the respiratory tract, abnormally dehydrated and thick mucus impedes normal mucociliary clearance creating a favorable environment for various organisms infect and prosper with colonies. Due to persistent mucus, the airways are colonized with several pathogens which leads to the accumulation of inflammatory mediators and increases inflammation [11]. At early stages of life, the most common bacteria detected in the sputum are *Staphylococcus aureus* and *Hemophilus influenzae*, contrary to this *Pseudomonas aeruginosa* is the most prevalent bacteria during the second and third decade of life [12]. *Pseudomonas aeruginosa*, *Burkholderia cepacia* complex, and methicillin-resistant *Staphylococcus aureus* are known to be associated with CF morbidity and mortality [13]. Persistent productive cough, breathlessness, wheeze, to begin with, leads to chronic lung infections, recurrent sinusitis and decreased exercise tolerance. Vicious cycles of infection, inflammation and mucus build-up not only cause multiple pulmonary exacerbations but slowly damage respiratory airways culminating into bronchiectasis. In later stage complications like organized pneumonia, atelectasis, hemoptysis, pneumothorax, pulmonary hypertension, chronic hypoxic and hypercapnic respiratory failure and cor pulmonale may occur [14, 15].

Abdominal manifestations of CF arise early in the course of the disease and have a severe impact on the quality of life of the patients. Dehydrated, concentrated pancreatic juices in CF patients cause a progressive obstruction and acute and chronic inflammation leading to parenchymal injury terminating into pancreatic insufficiency [16]. Clinical symptoms of pancreatic insufficiency include greasy

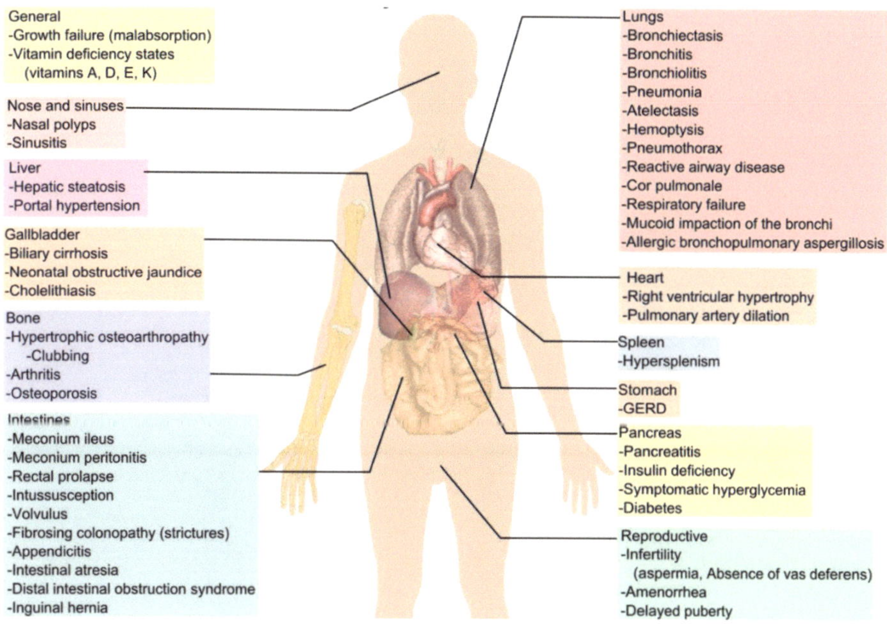

Figure 2.
Clinical presentation of cystic fibrosis (credit wikimedia.org.png).

stools, flatulence, abdominal bloating, and poor weight gain. The CF liver disease is characterized by the hyper-viscous bile causing obstructive cholangitis initially leading to focal biliary fibrosis and subsequently to biliary multinodular cirrhosis and portal hypertension [17]. Gastrointestinal manifestations of CF occur due to pancreatic insufficiency, thickened intestinal secretions, undigested food remnants, poor motility, and fecal stasis with resultant impaction of mucofeculent material in the distal ileum and right colon presented as meconium ileus in the newborn and distal intestinal obstruction syndrome in the post-neonatal life. Manifestations of CF extend beyond respiratory and gastro-intestinal symptoms to practically every system of the body as shown in **Figure 2**. A peculiar manifestation of CF that defies systemic boundaries, however, is CF-related diabetes (CFRD) that involves characteristics of both types of diabetes, that is, decreased secretion of insulin seen in type 1 due to scarring of the pancreas and decreased sensitivity to insulin seen in type 2 [18]. Incidence of CFRD increases with age and symptoms like unexplained weight loss, tiredness, increased thirst and micturition and sometimes decline in lung function can start in some patients in childhood itself. Microvascular complications like diabetic nephropathy, neuropathy and retinopathy are known to happen in untreated patients. Oral glucose tolerance test is a gold standard to detect the condition and should be performed at the age of 10 and yearly thereafter to diagnose and manage it at an early stage [19].

4. Diagnosis of cystic fibrosis

With the advent in diagnostic modalities, the CF is now diagnosed in newborns unlike a few decades ago when symptoms of CF and sometimes life-threatening CF complications prompted diagnostic procedures. However, even today false negative screening tests, migration, mild form of the disease and late presentation lets the condition undiagnosed until in the adulthood. Screening tests to clinch the diagnosis of CF at the earliest stage are offered at various levels. Carrier testing

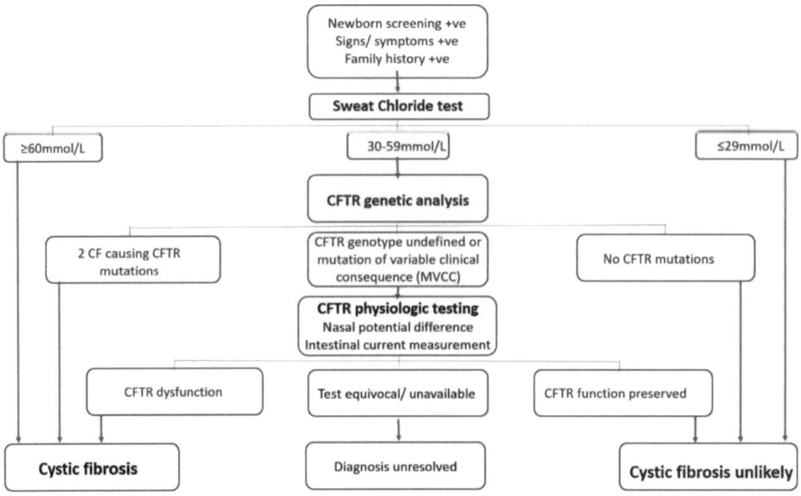

Figure 3.
Diagnosis of cystic fibrosis.

with blood or buccal mucosa analysis for common mutations in the CFTR gene is indicated in people who wants to have children and have a relative affected with the CF. Antenatal testing involves chorionic biopsy or amniocentesis for similar genetic analysis and is offered to when partners are known carriers of the disease. Newborn screening involves testing immunoreactive trypsinogen (IRT) in heel prick blood which is increased in CF due to obstructed pancreatic ductus [20]. Raised IRT mandates sweat test which measures chloride concentration in the sweat that allows categorization of patients into CF, 'CF unlikely' and 'intermediate' as shown in **Figure 3** prompting further evaluation by genetic testing in the intermediate category. In this, patients' blood is checked for the number of copies of CFTR gene affected with most common CF mutations- the inheritance of 2 copies of mutated gene confirms CF, while undefined CFTR genotype or mutation of variable clinical consequence requires CFTR physiologic testing to establish the diagnosis of CF [21]. Nasal potential difference evaluating salt transport in the nasal epithelial cells and intestinal current measurement may further help elucidating the diagnosis of CF in this group of patients [22].

5. Management of cystic fibrosis

Management of CF-related complications varies and is dependent on disease severity and rate of progression and as a result, treatment is highly individualized.

As the progression of lung disease has significant prognostic implications for patients with CF, treatment of lung disease is one of the cornerstones of CF treatment. Airway clearance is a key element of treatment and starts at birth or as soon as the patient is diagnosed. Airway clearance can be assisted by positive expiratory pressure devices and airway high-frequency chest wall oscillation techniques and should be performed daily (more frequently with advancing disease or during exacerbations) [23]. Airway clearance is assisted by treatments aimed at reducing the viscoelasticity of the mucous as thinner secretions are easier to expectorate. These involve nebulized treatment in the form of b-agonists, 3–6% hypertonic saline and dornase alpha as well as adequate levels of hydration [23, 24].

Preventing and controlling lung infections is central to the management of CF. Antibiotic regimes aim to prevent or treat exacerbations and to eradicate newly isolated pathogens. First isolation of gram-negative pathogens such as *Pseudomonas aeruginosa* should be prompt and attempt of eradication. Several eradications protocols including oral (typically ciprofloxacin) and inhaled antibiotics (typically tobramycin or colomycin) are available but details are beyond the scope of this chapter [25]. Prophylactic antibiotics aim to prevent or delay exacerbations, may be oral or inhaled and are used in conjunction with airway clearance techniques. They have been shown to reduce the frequency of exacerbations.

Pulmonary Exacerbations of CF include a combination of clinical symptoms, decline in lung function and oxygenation as well as rise of markers of inflammation. They are treated by a combination of antibiotic treatment, enhanced airway clearance and chest physiotherapy and supportive care as needed which may include oxygen supplementation or nutritional support. More severe exacerbations or exacerbations caused by more virulent and antibiotic-resistant pathogens will require intravenous antibiotics and a longer course of at least two weeks [24].

Haemoptysis and spontaneous pneumothorax are common complications of CF-related lung disease. Haemoptysis is often related to an infective exacerbation and treatment may be controlled with conservative measures such as treating the underlying infection and may require bronchial artery embolization or even lung resection. Repeated episodes of significant haemoptysis not controlled by embolization may be an indication for lung transplantation [26].

Treatment of gastrointestinal manifestations of CF includes treatment of pancreatic insufficiency and management of CF-related diabetes as well as prevention and treatment of intestinal blockage. Pancreatic insufficiency is treated with pancreatic enzyme replacement as well as nutritional support with high-calorie fat diet, vitamin supplementation and sodium chloride supplementation. Intestinal blockage prevention and treatment requires oral hydration, osmotic laxatives and hyperosmolar contrast enemas as needed [27, 28].

CF is a multisystem disease and therefore patients may also require treatment of other organs and systems such as complications from sinuses, urogenital complications as well as metabolic disorders such as reduced bone mineral density.

5.1 CFTR modulators – targeted treatment in CF disease

In recent years targeted therapy in the form of CFTR modulators has revolutionized the treatment of patients with CF. Oral, small molecules were developed that target the CFTR protein and have proven to be clinically successful in correcting the defect of the CFTR protein in vivo [29]. They are extremely efficacious and are transforming the care of patients living with CF - a chronic, progressive, multiorgan disease- in an unprecedented way. A detailed description of CFTR modulators is beyond the scope of this chapter. The first CFTR modulator -ivacaftor- was suitable for a relatively small percentage of patients with CF. There are currently four single or combination therapies available (with more being investigated) and they have revolutionized the management of patients with CF. Numerous CFTR modulators are currently being tested as well as gene engineering techniques aimed directly at the different mutations of the CF gene [30].

5.2 Lung transplantation in patients with CF

CF is a chronic progressive disease. Patients gradually develop structural changes in the lung parenchyma such as bronchiectasis. As the lung disease progresses the frequency of exacerbation increases as well as the likelihood of complications such as pneumothoraces and haemoptysis both of which are associated with advanced disease. Patients eventually develop respiratory failure. In these cases, lung transplantation presents a definitive treatment. Patients with reduced lung function (expressed as an FEV1 of <30% predicted), increasing frequency of exacerbations and/or increase in symptom burden as well as patients with life-threatening haemoptysis not controlled by embolization or with persistent recurrent pneumothorax should be considered for lung transplantation. Median survival after lung transplantation remains modest (7–8 years), however, it improves the quality of life and prognosis of patients with end-stage lung disease [26].

6. Conclusion

CF is a chronic, progressive, multiorgan disease caused by different mutations of the gene responsible for the CFTR protein. The involvement of lung disease is central in the clinical manifestations of the disease and carries significant prognostic implications for patients with CF. Early diagnosis and aggressive management with airway clearance and antibiotic treatment of lung disease as well as vigorous management of extrapulmonary complications have significantly improved the quality of life and survival of patients with CF. Lung transplantation remains a definitive treatment in patients with end-stage lung disease. However, the management of CF disease has entered an exciting era with CFTR modulators targeting the defective CFTR protein and have revolutionized the management and prognosis of CF.

Future studies are looking at gene engineering to target CFTR gene mutations which will hopefully provide new therapeutic targets.

Author details

Prashant N. Mohite* and Vicky Gerovasili
Royal Brompton and Harefield NHS Foundation Trust, United Kingdom

*Address all correspondence to: p.mohite@rbht.nhs.uk

References

[1] Hodson M, Geddes D, Bush A, eds. (2012). *Cystic Fibrosis* (3rd ed.). London: Hodder Arnold. p. 3. ISBN 978-1-4441-1369-3.

[2] Andersen DH. Cystic fibrosis of the pancreas and its relation to celiac disease: a clinical and pathologic study. Am J Dis Child. 1938;56(2):344-399.

[3] Di Sant'agnese PA, Drling RC, Perera GA, Shea E. Abnormal electrolyte composition of sweat in cystic fibrosis of the pancreas; clinical significance and relationship to the disease. Pediatrics. 1953 Nov;12(5):549-563.

[4] Tsui LC, Buchwald M. Biochemical and molecular genetics of cystic fibrosis. Adv Hum Genet. 1991;20:153-266, 311-2.

[5] The history, and the future, of cystic fibrosis | Royal Brompton & Harefield NHS Foundation Trust (rbht.nhs.uk) assessed on 27/01/2021.

[6] Korst RJ, McElvaney NG, Chu CS, Rosenfeld MA, Mastrangeli A, Hay J, Brody SL, Eissa NT, Danel C, Jaffe HA, et al. Gene therapy for the respiratory manifestations of cystic fibrosis. Am J Respir Crit Care Med. 1995 Mar;151 (3 Pt 2):S75–S87.

[7] Crystal RG, McElvaney NG, Rosenfeld MA, Chu CS, Mastrangeli A, Hay JG, Brody SL, Jaffe HA, Eissa NT, Danel C. Administration of an adenovirus containing the human CFTR cDNA to the respiratory tract of individuals with cystic fibrosis. Nat Genet. 1994 Sep;8(1):42-51.

[8] Vankeerberghen A, Cuppens H, Cassiman JJ. The cystic fibrosis transmembrane conductance regulator: an intriguing protein with pleiotropic functions. J Cyst Fibros. 2002 Mar;1(1):13-29.

[9] Reisin IL, Prat AG, Abraham EH, Amara JF, Gregory RJ, Ausiello DA, Cantiello HF. The cystic fibrosis transmembrane conductance regulator is a dual ATP and chloride channel. J Biol Chem. 1994 Aug 12;269(32):20584-20591.

[10] Lao O, Andrés AM, Mateu E, Bertranpetit J, Calafell F. Spatial patterns of cystic fibrosis mutation spectra in European populations. Eur J Hum Genet. 2003 May;11(5):385-394.

[11] Bhatt JM. Treatment of pulmonary exacerbations in cystic fibrosis. Eur Respir Rev. 2013 Sep 1;22(129):205-216.

[12] Lyczak JB, Cannon CL, Pier GB. Lung infections associated with cystic fibrosis. Clin Microbiol Rev 2002;15:194-222.

[13] Navarro J, Rainisio M, Harms HK, Hodson ME, Koch C, Mastella G, Strandvik B, McKenzie SG. Factors associated with poor pulmonary function: cross-sectional analysis of data from the ERCF. European Epidemiologic Registry of Cystic Fibrosis. Eur Respir J. 2001 Aug;18(2):298-305.

[14] Flume PA, Mogayzel Jr PJ, Robinson KA, Rosenblatt RL, Quittell L, Marshall BC. Clinical Practice Guidelines for Pulmonary Therapies Committee; Cystic Fibrosis Foundation Pulmonary Therapies Committee. Cystic fibrosis pulmonary guidelines: pulmonary complications: hemoptysis and pneumothorax. Am J Respir Crit Care Med 2010; 182 (03) 298-306.

[15] Garcia B, Flume PA. Pulmonary Complications of Cystic Fibrosis. Semin Respir Crit Care Med. 2019 Dec;40(6):804-809.

[16] Sathe MN, Freeman AJ. Gastrointestinal, Pancreatic, and

Hepatobiliary Manifestations of Cystic Fibrosis. Pediatr Clin North Am. 2016 Aug;63(4):679-698.

[17] Gabel ME, Galante GJ, Freedman SD. Gastrointestinal and Hepatobiliary Disease in Cystic Fibrosis. Semin Respir Crit Care Med. 2019 Dec;40(6):825-841.

[18] Moheet A, Moran A. CF-related diabetes: Containing the metabolic miscreant of cystic fibrosis. Pediatr Pulmonol. 2017 Nov;52(S48):S37-S43.

[19] Lek N, Acerini CL. Cystic fibrosis related diabetes mellitus - diagnostic and management challenges. Curr Diabetes Rev. 2010 Jan;6(1):9-16.

[20] Coverstone AM, Ferkol TW. Early Diagnosis and Intervention in Cystic Fibrosis: Imagining the Unimaginable. Front Pediatr. 2021 Jan 11;8:608821.

[21] Farrell PM, White TB, Ren CL, Hempstead SE, Accurso F, Derichs N, Howenstine M, McColley SA, Rock M, Rosenfeld M, Sermet-Gaudelus I, Southern KW, Marshall BC, Sosnay PR. Diagnosis of Cystic Fibrosis: Consensus Guidelines from the Cystic Fibrosis Foundation. J Pediatr. 2017 Feb;181S:S4-S15.e1.

[22] Minso R, Schulz A, Dopfer C, Alfeis N, Barneveld AV, Makartian-Gyulumyan L, Hansen G, Junge S, Müller C, Ringshausen FCC, Sauer-Heilborn A, Stanke F, Stolpe C, Tamm S, Welte T, Dittrich AM, Tümmler B. Intestinal current measurement and nasal potential difference to make a diagnosis of cases with inconclusive *CFTR* genetics and sweat test. BMJ Open Respir Res. 2020 Oct;7(1):e000736.

[23] Mogayzel PJ Jr, Naureckas ET, Robinson KA, et al. Pulmonary Clinical Practice Guidelines Committee. Cystic fibrosis pulmonary guidelines. Chronic medications for maintenance of lung health. Am J Respir Crit Care Med 2013; 187: 680-689

[24] Robinson M, Regnis JA, Bailey DL, et al. Efect of hypertonic saline, amiloride, and cough on mucociliary clearance in patients with cystic fbrosis. Am J Respir Crit Care Med. 1996;153:1503-1509.

[25] Döring G, Flume P, Heijerman H, Elborn JS; Consensus Study Group. Treatment of lung infection in patients with cystic fibrosis: current and future strategies. J Cyst Fibros 2012; 11: 461-479

[26] Weill D, Benden C, Corris PA, Dark JH, Davis RD, Keshavjee S, Lederer DJ, Mulligan MJ, Patterson GA, Singer LG, Snell GI, Verleden GM, Zamora MR, Glanville AR. A consensus document for the selection of lung transplant candidates: 2014--an update from the Pulmonary Transplantation Council of the International Society for Heart and Lung Transplantation. J Heart Lung Transplant. 2015 Jan;34(1):1-15.

[27] Colombo C, Ellemunter H, Houwen R, et al. Guidelines for the diagnosis and management of distal intestinal obstruction syndrome in cystic fbrosis patients. J Cyst Fibros. 2011;10(Suppl 2):S24-8. 27.

[28] Stern RC, Eisenberg JD, Wagener JS, et al. A comparison of the efcacy and tolerance of pancrelipase and placebo in the treatment of steatorrhea in cystic fbrosis patients with clinical exocrine pancreatic insuffciency. Am J Gastroenterol. 2000;95:1932-1938.

[29] Ramos KJ, Pilewski JM, Taylor-Cousar JL. Challenges in the use of highly effective modulator treatment for cystic fibrosis. J Cyst Fibros. 2021 Jan 30:S1569-1993(21)00026-6.

[30] Rafeeq MM, Murad HAS. Cystic fibrosis: current therapeutic targets and future approaches. J Transl Med 2017 Apr 27;15(1):84

Chapter 2

Cystic Fibrosis-Related Diabetes (CFRD)

Manfred Ballmann

Abstract

Cystic fibrosis-related diabetes (CFRD) is the most frequent comorbidity in CF. The prevalence is age-dependent and abnormalities in/of glucose homeostasis start early in life. As CFRD has an impact on pulmonary function and life expectancy, early diagnosis and treatment is mandatory. Screening is needed because initially, most patients with CFRD do not show any typical symptoms of diabetes. The question of which screening method gets the best results is still under discussion. For treatment insulin is recommended but a relevant percentage of patients do not use it, and even if insulin is used, there is no consensus on what the best insulin regime in the case of CFRD is. Recently, oral antidiabetic drugs were shown to be as effective and safe as insulin in the initial treatment of CFRD. This treatment might reduce the additional treatment burden for patients with CFRD. The best way to monitor CFRD is also under discussion (HbA1c and/or continuous glucose monitoring; CGM). The threshold of HbA1c might be lower than for other types of diabetes. As patients with CF become older, the duration of CFRD will also increase and typical diabetes complications will occur. So far, these are mainly microvascular complications. The new CFTR modulators might influence not only pulmonary function but potentially also glucose homeostasis.

Keywords: CFRD, epidemiology, diagnosis, screening, treatment, CFTR modulators

1. Introduction

CF is a multi-organ disease that also affects the exocrine and endocrine pancreas [1]. CFRD is a discrete entity of type 3 Diabetes mellitus, displaying aspects from both type 1 Diabetes mellitus and type 2 Diabetes mellitus. It is the most frequent comorbidity in CF involving around 31% of CF patients older than 18 years [2] and up to more than 40% in those older than 30 years [3]. It results from involvement of the endocrine pancreatic function and is the end stage of early onset impaired glucose homeostasis [4]. Today, additional CFRD is still a risk factor for decreased pulmonary function but no longer for increased mortality [3]. In the past, an increased mortality, in part depending on sex and severe CFTR mutation, was observed [5]. Several aspects of the disease's pathophysiology are not yet completely understood [6], but some new insights might help to understand the process [7]. Clinically, there is a need for screening since earlier prospective studies regarding CFRD showed that most CF patients exhibited no clinical signs of hyperglycemia at the time they were diagnosed with CFRD by oral glucose tolerance tests (OGTTs) [8]. The advantages and disadvantages of different screening approaches will be discussed. Even after diagnosis, there is some discussion on how to treat patients with CFRD diagnosed by screening. Guidelines recommended insulin treatment [9] but registry data from the US [2] and Europe [10] showed that a relevant proportion of CF patients with CFRD are not treated with daily insulin. Alternative treatment options might be needed, and a recent study demonstrated that oral antidiabetic drugs are not inferior to insulin regarding HbA1c over 2 years after CFRD was diagnosed by annual OGTT screening [11]. Upcoming CFTR modulator treatment is an interesting area regarding glucose homeostasis and CFRD. The results of two small case studies [12, 13] on CF patients treated with ivacaftor imply that there is a possibility that CFTR modulation might also influence insulin secretion. Additionally, a registry study showed a trend to a reduced prevalence of CFRD in those treated with ivacaftor for a longer time [14]. In another case study with five patients (F508 del homozygous) treated with lumacaftor/ivacaftor, no consistent effect on glucose tolerance or insulin secretion was observed [15]. Overall, there are a number of important aspects of CFRD, from its pathophysiology to screening, diagnosis, treatment, best methods of follow-up, and new perspectives with CFTR modulator treatment options.

2. CFRD and epidemiology

2.1 Prevalence and incidence and risk factors

In 1994, a first study reporting the prevalence of CFRD was published [16]. Prevalence was 14.7% in all Danish CF patients. More recent data from the CFF patient registry showed an age-dependent prevalence from around 2% in those younger than 10 years up to around 40–50% in adults [2]. The prevalence is in the same range as reported from Germany (**Table 1**) [17] as a European country. The prevalence varies between different European countries based on a recent report of the ECFS patient registry [18]. While diabetes prevalence has risen, incidence has fallen significantly: from 4 cases per 100 patient-years during the 1998–2002 interval to 2.7 cases per 100 patient-years between 2003 and 2008, representing a 40% decrease in the number of diabetes diagnoses in the US [3]. In a longitudinal study from the UK, the incidence was 3.5% (observation period 1996–2005) [19].

Severe genotype, pancreatic insufficiency, and female gender remain considerable intrinsic risk factors for early acquisition of CFRD [18]. In a large prospective study with 1093 patients, impaired fasting glucose, impaired glucose tolerance, and indeterminate glucose tolerance were all predictors of future CFRD [20] .

2.2 Sex differences and mortality

An increased mortality used to be described mainly for female CF patients with CFRD [21]. Mortality rate decreased from 1992–1997 to 2003–2008 in females from

Diabetes in CF	0–5 years	6–11 yeas	12–17 years	18–29 years	30–39 years	>40 years
Diabetes	0.1	1.2	11.1	21.6	32.0	46.6
Of these CFRD	0.0	100	86.7	96.5	94.5	94.3
Of these not CFRD	0.1	0.0	13.3	3.6	5.5	5.7

Adapted from table 17 and table 18 [17].

Table 1.
Frequency in % of CF patients with diabetes in 2018.

6.9 to 3.2 deaths per 100 patient-years and in male subjects from 6.5 to 3.8 deaths per 100 patient-years. There was no longer a sex difference in mortality [3]. A follow-up study (2008–2012) from the same CF center reported that there still was a sex difference in adults, but only in severe genotypes with higher prevalence of CFRD, resulting in an increased mortality in females [22]. Consequently, there is still a discussion about the gender influence on CFRD and survival.

2.3 Genetics

Since the CF gene was detected, there has been the question of a CFTR mutation/mutation class-related risk for CFRD or whether there are other mutations outside of the CFTR gene that may modify the risk of developing CFRD.

In a longitudinal study from the UK, CFTR mutation classes I and II were shown to increase the risk of CFRD independently of other known risk factors [19]. A more recent study reported the risk for CFRD and mortality in adults studied in the years 2008–2012 [22]. CFRD was associated with increased mortality independently of mutation category (mild or severe) [22].

A study looking for CFRD frequency in different age groups and the influence of mutation classes of the CFTR gene found that the prevalence of CFRD increased with age from 2.6% in patients <18 years to 22.1% in patients 18 years or older in those homozygous for group II (including del phen 508, the most frequent CFTR mutation) mutations. It was only 1.5% in patients 18 years or older in group IV/any CFTR mutations [23]. In general, group IV mutations are less severe than class II mutations and this results also in a low risk for CFRD. If CFRD as a complication of CF has developed, there is still an increased mortality risk even in mild mutation classes (e.g., CFTR mutation class IV), but the risk for developing CFRD is higher in severe CFTR mutation classes (e.g., CFTR mutation class I or II).

2.3.1 Genetic modifiers

The frequency of HLA types related to type 1 or type 2 diabetes were in the same range in CF patients with or without diabetes. There was also no difference in frequency compared to normal population [23]. As for other comorbidities, there are also modifiers for CFRD. Susceptibility to CFRD is at least in part determined by variants at SLC26A9 and at four loci associated with type 2 diabetes in the general population [24]. In a very recent study, a wide overlap with genetic modifiers of type 2 diabetes was described [25]. This might allow for a stratification of CFRD screening. Those with less risk depending on CFTR mutation classes and modifier genes might be screened starting at an older age and less frequently than those with a high risk for CFRD.

3. CFRD and pathophysiology

The mechanism of how diabetes develops in CF is not yet completely understood. Difficult access to animal models and human pancreatic tissue may contribute to this situation. Two recent reviews focused on the pathogenesis of CFRD [26, 27]. Insulin secretion is reduced even with normal OGTT and this is observed even in kids [28]. Insulin sensitivity is not or only minimally impaired apart from severe infections or systemic glucocorticoid treatment [29]. An often-discussed question concerned the possible existence of a direct influence of CFTR on α or β-cells. In an elegant study, murine models of β-cell CFTR deletion and human pancreas and islets from controls and CF patients were used [7]. There were some important results: (1) In the murine cell model, CFTR did not affect β-cell function. (2) In human islets, nearly no expression of CFTR mRNA was detected. (3) Additionally, there was no CFTR protein or electrical activity. (4) The secretion of islet hormones (insulin and glucagon) was in the normal range and only minimal changes in important islet-regulatory transcripts were detected. (5) As a consequence of inflammation, only 35% of β-cell area was conserved and the other part of the islet was compounded by immune infiltration. Overall, CFRD seems to be a consequence of beta-cell loss, accompanied by inflammation of the islets. There is no reason to think that CFTR mutations directly cause islet dysfunction [7].

4. CFRD and diagnosis

4.1 Screening, initial symptoms, and outcome

As there are usually no typical diabetes-related symptoms [8], there is a need to screen for CFRD. Guidelines recommended a regular oral glucose tolerance test (OGTT) for screening [9]. Annual screening should start at the age of 10 years, as recommended in the US and by the ECFS, or at 12 years, as recommended in the UK. Because OGTT is time-consuming for patients and CF center staff, there is some interest in more comfortable alternative methods. The screening rate with OGTT in CF is nowhere near the recommendations in guidelines. In median, only 61.3% of CF patients aged 10–17 years and only 32.8% of adults were screened by OGTT in the US [2]. Nevertheless, it is possible to increase the rate of screening by OGTT, as shown from a program in a pediatric CF center that increased its annual screening rate for outpatients from 45% to 71% [30].

In a registry study, it has recently been reported that CF centers that screen more frequently for CFRD detected CFRD earlier and that those that screened less often had a faster decrease in pulmonary function [31]. This supports the view that screening for CFRD is an important tool to optimize CF care.

4.1.1 HbA1c for screening

HbA1c is quickly collected and simple to measure, which makes it a comfortable test for both patients and CF center staff. To reduce the need for OGTT, the question was whether HbA1c was able to identify those patients at risk for CFRD. However, because of low sensitivity to detect CFRD, HbA1c has not been recommended as a screening tool for CFRD [32] for many years. This has recently become controversial. If a low HbA1c (<5.5%) as threshold was used to identify CF patients with CFRD, the sensitivity covered a wide range from 93% [33] to only 78% [34]. As of now, there is not enough evidence that HbA1c is a reliable tool to screen for CFRD.

4.1.2 Different OGTT methods

To make OGTT more comfortable for patients and staff, different modifications of the OGTT procedure were investigated. A shorter sample time (1 h) [35, 36] was discussed, as well as a lower glucose load (50 g) [37]. Both approaches need evaluation in a larger cohort. So far, standard (WHO) OGTT is still recommended.

4.1.3 Continuous glucose monitoring (CGM)

Another way to uncover impaired glucose homeostasis and CFRD even earlier than using OGTT is CGM. OGTTs were compared with 6 days of CGM in detecting glucose disturbance in 30 CF patients (age: 10–18 years). CGM identified glucose changes that had been missed by OGTT. This might help to initiate treatment of glucose disturbance before CFRD is diagnosed [38]. However, since even OGTT is only rarely used in many CF centers there is no reason to expect that the more sophisticated CGM will be used more frequently.

4.1.4 OGTT performance and diagnostic criteria

- OGTT: Glucose 1.75 g/kg body weight in 250–300 ml water max 75 g glucose drinking in 5 min

- Performed after >8 h of fasting in the morning.

- No physical activity during the test.

- Often the OGTT is done during the annual assessment. No other investigations during the OGTT (such as an ultrasound) are allowed.

- Blood glucose is measured before (0 min) and 60 min and 120 min after drinking the glucose load.

5. CFRD and treatment

5.1 Treatment

Disturbance of glucose homeostasis starts early in life, CFRD being the end stage [4]. This opens the discussion on the best time to start treatment even before CFRD is diagnosed by OGTT. Insulin is the only recommended treatment. This should be accompanied by an education program and dietary advice. Despite recommendations, insulin is used only in around 75% of all CFRD patients all over the world [2, 17, 40].

5.1.1 Insulin

Insulin is the recommended treatment for CFRD. There are two problems with this recommendation. (1) A relevant percentage of CFRD patients do not use insulin (see **Table 2**). This is the case in the US [2], the UK [41], and Germany [17] at least, as the national registers documented. All these are registries sponsored by CF organizations. Data from a German/Austrian general diabetes registry [42] that collects data from both CFRD patients and type 1 and 2 diabetes patients have shown that only 77% of CFRD patients were on insulin [40]. There might be several reasons for this. First of all, most patients do not realize symptoms of hyperglycemia early in the course of CFRD [8]. Secondly, CF treatment is an enormous burden for adult CF patients and families [43] as well as for children with CF. They spent 74 min a day with treatment, compared to type 1 diabetes with 56 min and asthma with 6 min [44]. Perhaps they like to avoid this additional burden of insulin treatment. (2) The optimal insulin regime is not defined and different regimes are in use. This includes long-term once-daily insulin, intensified insulin treatment several times a day, or an insulin pump with continuous insulin and pushes with meals. The more intensive insulin treatment with a pump is less in use, at least in adolescents and young adults, compared to type 1 diabetes patients in the same age range [45]. In adult CFRD patients treated with insulin, the mean daily dose was not different to matched type 1 or type 2 diabetes patients [46].

	Blood glucose mmol/l (mg/dl)		
	Start	**60 min**	**120 min**
Normal glucose tolerance (NGT)	<5·6 (100)	<11·1 (200)	<7·8 (140)
Fasting hyperglycemia (FH)	>5·6 (100) and <7·0 (126)	<11·1 (200)	<7·8 (140)
Impaired glucose tolerance (IGT)	<7·0 (126)	<11·1 (200)	>7·8 (140) <11·1 (200)
Indeterminate glycemia (INDET)	<7·0 (126)	>11·1 (200)	<7·8 (140)
Diabetes (CFRD) without FH	<7·0 (126)	–	>11·1 (200)
CFRD with FH	≥7·0 (126)	–	>11·1 (200)

Adapted from [39].

Table 2.
Classification of glucose tolerance.

One single optimal insulin regime for all CFRD patients does not exist, since individual adjustment to medical needs and patients' options is required. The treatment of CFRD is a team approach including dieticians, diabetologists, psychologists, and the CF physician.

5.1.2 Oral antidiabetic drugs

Oral antidiabetic drugs have been used in CFRD for many years [47]. The group of sulfonylurea (glibenclamide) had some disadvantages. They showed inhibitions of CFTR Cl channels in vitro [48–50]. The non-sulfonylurea hypoglycemic agent repaglinide showed only a weak inhibition of CFTR Cl channels [51]. In 2001, a study was published that showed postprandial effects of premeal insulin lispro and premeal repaglinide on postprandial glucose levels in humans. Glucose decreased (peak, 2 h and 5 h AUC) with insulin lispro, and glucose decreased with repaglinide only 5 h AUC. Insulin secretion (5 h AUC) increased only with insulin lispro [52]. In the latest Cochrane review regarding the use of oral antidiabetic drugs in CFRD, published in 2016, it was concluded that controlled prospective studies are needed [53]. There are two prospective randomized controlled trials comparing the effects of insulin versus repaglinide in patients with newly diagnosed CFRD [11, 54]. In a 12-month trial, there was a significant increase in BMI only in the insulin group. Comparing the insulin to the repaglinide group, there was no significant difference in BMI, HbA1c, or pulmonary function changes over the study period [54]. In the other study over 24 months, there was no difference between the groups (insulin and repaglinide) regarding HbA1c, BMI, and pulmonary function. It was concluded from that study that at least a subgroup of patients with newly diagnosed CFRD can be treated initially with oral antidiabetic drugs [11]. This might be an option for those who refuse insulin due to the additional treatment burden (**Table 3**).

Indication therapy in case of CFRD	0–5 years	6–11 yeas	12–17 years	18–29 years	30–39 years	>40 years
Insulin	100	72.7	64.0	67.6	76.9	75.7
Oral antidiabetics	0	9.1	11.0	9.3	9.3	8.8
Dietary measures	0	27.3	39.0	21	25	23.3

Adapted from table 22 and table 23 [17].

Table 3.
Frequency in % of CF patients with indication therapies related to diabetes in 2018.

5.1.3 Diet

The well-known diet restrictions and advice for type 1 or type 2 diabetes are not transferable to CFRD. In CFRD, the patients need a high-caloric nutrition, in contrast to what is recommended in other types of diabetes. Therefore, a dietician trained in CFRD is needed to support the patient with detailed information regarding nutrition in the special situation of CFRD [55].

5.2 Treatment monitoring

5.2.1 HbA1c

HbA1c is not recommended to diagnose CFRD (see Section 4.1.1.). The situation is different for monitoring CFRD. HbA1c is used to monitor glycemic control in CFRD. In CFRD, the target value for HbA1c should be lower than in type 1 diabetes, because in CFRD mean plasma glucose does not correlate with HbA1c [56]. This is, for example, incorporated in the Australian Standards of Care for CFRD [57]. Adults with CFRD have a significantly lower HbA1c value compared to type 1 diabetes adults (6.8% vs. 7.9%) [58]. How low HbA1c values should be to prevent long-term diabetic comorbidities like microangiopathies (see also Section 6.1) is unknown.

5.2.2 CGM

A more strict control of glucose homeostasis with insulin treatment is achievable with CGM and is accompanied by an improved clinical outcome [59]. This requires the cooperation of the entire CFRD team and particularly the support by a diabetologist.

In general, adherence to diabetes care guidelines (ADA/CFF) is suboptimal [40] and improvement is urgently needed.

6. CFRD and complications

6.1 Microvascular complications

With decreased mortality, CF patients spend more years living with CFRD. Today, CF patients tend to develop microvascular complications, much like patients with type 1 or type 2 diabetes [60]. In long-standing CFRD (>10 years) with fasting hyperglycemia, 14% of patients had microalbuminuria and 16% had retinopathy [61]. The percentage of patients with hypertension was lower in adult CFRD patients while the percentage of patients suffering from nephropathy was higher compared to type 1 and 2 diabetes [58]. These data underline the need for routine screening for CFRD complications.

6.1.1 Retinal complications

More sophisticated eye investigations demonstrated changes at the retina level.

Screening for this kind of complication should be also mandatory [62]. Percentage of patients with retinopathy did not differ between adults with CFRD and type 1 or type 2 diabetes [58].

6.1.2 Macrovascular complications

Macrovascular complications have not been described so far. However, with increasing duration of CFRD in older CF patients, this kind of complication has to be expected. Even microvascular complications develop later in CFRD than in other types of diabetes.

6.2 Risk for hyperglycemia

The risk for acute severe hyperglycemia exists but the condition is very rare [63]. Most CFRD patients do not develop a ketoacidosis. This might be related to residual insulin secretion and glucagon counter regulation. Hyperglycemia measured by HbA1c is a risk factor for mortality. In a prospective observational study, a HbA1c ≥ 6.5% was associated with a threefold increased risk of death [64]. Measuring HbA1c is mandatory and it should be kept in mind that the target value is lower than in type 1 or type 2 diabetes (see also Section 5.2.1).

6.3 Risk for hypoglycemia

The detected frequency of hypoglycemia is higher with CGM than with OGTT [65]. There is no prognostic relevance of hypoglycemia during OGT for later development of CFRD [66]. In general, it seems that the risk of hypoglycemia is not different from other types of diabetes and instruction on how to handle CFRD in daily life should address this risk.

7. CFRD and special situations

7.1 Pregnancy

With improved clinical course of CF and improved life expectancy, more female CF patients want to become pregnant. According to the UK guidelines [55], there are four groups.

- CFRD and IGT: optimized diabetes control and needs to be referred to a specialized diabetes team.
- NGT (tested in the last 3 months): OGT in first trimester and the next between week 24 and week 28.
- Unknown glycemic status: OGT before becoming pregnant, if possible.

7.2 Physical activity

With better clinical conditions, physical activities in all age groups of CF patients increased. Patients with CFRD should exercise and be educated about the risk of hypoglycemia, like other diabetic patients. CFRD is no reason to stop physical activities.

8. CFRD and cystic fibrosis transmembrane regulator (CFTR) modulators

Since 2012, there is a new class of medication for CF patients on the market. These drugs are called “CFTR modulators.” They are CFTR mutation specific and are administered orally. This offers the chance that these drugs might affect different organs that are reached by the bloodstream. The regulation of glucose homeostasis is a complex process and CFTR modulators might interfere at different steps.

8.1 CFRD and ivacaftor

Ivacaftor is a CFTR potentiator and acts with gating mutations (e.g., G551D). It increases pulmonary function, weight, and quality of life (QoL) and decreases sweat chloride concentration [67].

In two siblings, insulin secretion and glucose AUC were measured during an OGTT before and 16 weeks after initiation of ivacaftor [12]. This paper described the beneficial effect of 4-month ivacaftor treatment on the pathologic OGTT of two patients with CF carrying the S549R gating mutation. This beneficial effect may be partially due to the increased earlier insulin secretion capacity [12]. Two other studies also reported an increase in insulin secretion after ivacaftor was initiated in CF patients with a gating mutation [68, 69]. As of now, reports have included only small numbers of patients and/or are uncontrolled studies. Sufficiently powered studies are still missing. In a registry study using data from the US and the UK with a follow-up of more than 5 years, a trend to a reduced prevalence of CFRD in ivacaftor-treated patients [14] was reported. If this observation will be corroborated in future studies, many CF patients would benefit from a postponed CFRD treatment burden.

8.2 CFRD and Ivacaftor/lumacaftor combination therapy

The combination therapy with ivacaftor/lumacaftor was administered to patients with the del F508 mutation [70]. The overall clinical effect regarding pulmonary function, weight, and QoL was low compared to ivacaftor in patients with a gating mutation [67]. Using CGM and OGTT to control glucose homeostasis in five patients after initiation of ivacaftor/lumacaftor treatment, glycemic abnormalities persisted [71]. A consistent impact of the combination of ivacaftor/lumacaftor on insulin secretion or glucose tolerance was not detected in five patients [15]. In a very recent article from France [72], the change of OGTT categories after 1 year of lumacaftor/ivacaftor treatment was described in an uncontrolled study design. The reported improvement, for example, from CFRD to IGT is within the range of the well-known high variability of OGTT results in CF patients [73]. It is not surprising that the combination treatment, which had less of an effect on clinical outcome in gating mutations compared to ivacaftor, has so far no proven effect on CFRD, even if only a small number of CF patients were investigated.

8.3 CFRD and outlook

The recently published results with a triple combination CFTR modulator therapy in patients with a del phen 508 allele are impressive regarding pulmonary function increase, sweat chloride decrease, and other outcomes [74]. With a highly clinically effective CFTR modulator treatment and a sufficient number of patients, the demonstration of a positive influence on glucose homeostasis in a prospective study seems realistic.

However, there is currently no evidence-based information that CFTR modulators have a relevant influence on the complex pathophysiology regarding glucose homeostasis.

9. Conclusions

CFRD is still a highly relevant comorbidity in CF. Nevertheless, there are many questions regarding its optimal handling from both patients' and physicians' point of view. CFRD is a team approach, which includes the CF team but also the diabetes team.

Adherence to all aspects of CFRD diagnosis and treatment is low and needs urgent efforts to increase.

As long as no better screening procedure is established, 2h of OGTT should be used annually as screening for CFRD.

Education regarding CFRD should include patients, families, physicians, and the entire team.

Treatment as recommended by guidelines prefers only insulin. The recently published controlled prospective trials may endorse the use of oral antidiabetic drugs, at least in a subgroup of patients.

Monitoring must include all the measurements that are recommended for other types of diabetes. HbA1c target value for treatment should be lower than in type 1 or 2 diabetes.

Typical microvascular complications are reported and patients should be regularly checked for these.

In future, the new and effective CFTR modulator therapies might also influence the prevalence of CFRD. In a perfect world, they might also improve glucose homeostasis in patients with CFRD and postpone CFRD entirely.

Conflict of interest

The authors declare no conflict of interest.

Author details

Manfred Ballmann
University Medicine Rostock, Rostock, Germany

*Address all correspondence to: manfred.ballmann@med.uni-rostock.de

References

[1] Elborn JS. Cystic fibrosis. Lancet. 2016;**388**(10059):2519-2531

[2] Annual Data Report 2018. Cystic Fibrosis Foundation Patient Registry. 2019. Available from: https://www.cff.org/Research/Researcher-Resources/Patient-Registry/2018-Patient-Registry-Annual-Data-Report.pdf

[3] Moran A et al. Cystic fibrosis-related diabetes: Current trends in prevalence, incidence, and mortality. Diabetes Care. 2009;**32**(9):1626-1631

[4] Yi Y et al. Abnormal glucose tolerance in infants and young children with cystic fibrosis. American Journal of Respiratory and Critical Care Medicine. 2016;**194**(8):974-980

[5] Chamnan P et al. Diabetes as a Determinant of Mortality in Cystic Fibrosis. Diabetes Care. 2009

[6] Moran A et al. Epidemiology, pathophysiology, and prognostic implications of cystic fibrosis-related diabetes: a technical review. Diabetes Care. 2010;**33**(12):2677-2683

[7] Hart NJ et al. Cystic fibrosis-related diabetes is caused by islet loss and inflammation. JCI Insight. 2018;**3**(8)

[8] Lanng S et al. Glucose tolerance in patients with cystic fibrosis: five year prospective study. BMJ. 1995;**311**(7006):655-659

[9] Moran A et al. Clinical care guidelines for cystic fibrosis-related diabetes: a position statement of the American Diabetes Association and a clinical practice guideline of the Cystic Fibrosis Foundation, endorsed by the Pediatric Endocrine Society. Diabetes Care. 2010;**33**(12):2697-2708

[10] ECFSPR Annual Report 2017. 2019 [cited 2020 1.2.2020]; Available from: https://www.ecfs.eu/sites/default/files/general-content-images/working-groups/ecfs-patient-registry/ECFSPR_Report2017_v1.3.pdf

[11] Ballmann M et al. Repaglinide versus insulin for newly diagnosed diabetes in patients with cystic fibrosis: a multicentre, open-label, randomised trial. The Lancet Diabetes and Endocrinology. 2018;**6**(2):114-121

[12] Tsabari R et al. CFTR potentiator therapy ameliorates impaired insulin secretion in CF patients with a gating mutation. Journal of Cystic Fibrosis. 2016;**15**(3):e25-e27

[13] Christian F et al. Sustained glycemic control with ivacaftor in cystic fibrosis-related diabetes. Journal of Investigative Medicine High Impact Case Reports;7:2019 2324709619842898

[14] Volkova N et al. Disease progression in patients with cystic fibrosis treated with ivacaftor. Journal of Cystic Fibrosis;7:2019 2324709619842898

[15] Thomassen JC et al. Effect of lumacaftor/ivacaftor on glucose metabolism and insulin secretion in Phe508del homozygous cystic fibrosis patients. Journal of Cystic Fibrosis. 2018;**17**(2):271-275

[16] Lanng S et al. Diabetes mellitus in Danish cystic fibrosis patients: Prevalence and late diabetic complications. Acta Paediatrica. 1994;**83**(1):72-77

[17] Annual report 2018. German Cystic Fibrosis Registry. 2019. Available from: https://www.muko.info/fileadmin/user_upload/angebote/qualitaetsmanagement/register/berichtsbaende/annual_report_2018.pdf

[18] Olesen HV et al. Cystic fibrosis related diabetes in Europe: Prevalence, risk factors and outcome. Journal of Cystic Fibrosis. 2019;**18**(6):874-878

[19] Adler AI et al. Genetic determinants and epidemiology of cystic fibrosis-related diabetes: Results from a British cohort of children and adults. Diabetes Care. 2008;**31**(9):1789-1794

[20] Schmid K et al. Predictors for future cystic fibrosis-related diabetes by oral glucose tolerance test. Journal of Cystic Fibrosis. 2014;**13**(1):80-85

[21] Milla CE, Billings J, Moran A. Diabetes is associated with dramatically decreased survival in female but not male subjects with cystic fibrosis. Diabetes Care. 2005;**28**(9):2141-2144

[22] Lewis C et al. Diabetes-related mortality in adults with cystic fibrosis role of genotype and sex. American Journal of Respiratory and Critical Care Medicine. 2015;**191**(2):194-200

[23] Lanng S et al. Diabetes mellitus in cystic fibrosis: Genetic and immunological markers. Acta Paediatrica. 1993;**82**(2):150-154

[24] Blackman SM et al. Genetic modifiers of cystic fibrosis-related diabetes. Diabetes. 2013;**62**(10):3627-3635

[25] Aksit MA et al. Genetic modifiers of cystic fibrosis-related diabetes have extensive overlap with type 2 diabetes and related traits. The Journal of Clinical Endocrinology and Metabolism. 2020;**105**(5):1-15

[26] Ode KL et al. New insights into cystic fibrosis-related diabetes in children. The Lancet Diabetes and Endocrinology. 2013;**1**(1):52-58

[27] Yoon JC. Evolving mechanistic views and emerging therapeutic strategies for cystic fibrosis-related diabetes. Journal of the Endocrine Society. 2017;**1**(11):1386-1400

[28] Lombardo F et al. Natural history of glucose tolerance, beta-cell function and peripheral insulin sensitivity in cystic fibrosis patients with fasting euglycemia. European Journal of Endocrinology. 2003;**149**(1):53-59

[29] Battezzati A et al. Identification of insulin secretory defects and insulin resistance during oral glucose tolerance test in a cohort of cystic fibrosis patients. European Journal of Endocrinology. 2011;**165**(1):69-76

[30] Kern AS et al. Improving screening for cystic fibrosis-related diabetes at a pediatric cystic fibrosis program. Pediatrics. 2013;**132**(2):e512-e518

[31] Franck Thompson E et al. The association of pediatric cystic fibrosis-related diabetes screening on clinical outcomes by center. Journal of Cystic Fibrosis. 2019;**40**(5):466-470

[32] Holl RW et al. HbA1c is not recommended as a screening test for diabetes in cystic fibrosis. Diabetes Care. 2000;**23**(1):126

[33] Lam GY et al. How reliable is your HbA1c test? Revisiting the use of HbA1c in cystic fibrosis-related diabetes (CFRD) screening. Journal of Cystic Fibrosis. 2019;**18**(2):e14-e15

[34] Tommerdahl KL et al. Screening for cystic fibrosis-related diabetes and prediabetes: Evaluating 1,5-anhydroglucitol, fructosamine, glycated albumin, and hemoglobin A1c. Pediatric Diabetes. 2019;**20**(8):1080-1086

[35] Sheikh S et al. Elevation of one hour plasma glucose during oral glucose tolerance testing. Pediatric Pulmonology. 2015;**50**(10):963-969

[36] Coriati A et al. Diagnosis of cystic fibrosis-related glucose abnormalities: Can we shorten the standard oral glucose tolerance test? Applied Physiology Nutrition and Metabolism. 2013;**38**(12):1254-1259

[37] Sheikh S et al. Abnormal glucose tolerance and the 50-gram glucose challenge test in cystic fibrosis. Journal of Cystic Fibrosis. 2020. DOI: 10.1016/j.jcf.2020.01.003

[38] Clemente Leon M et al. Oral glucose tolerance test and continuous glucose monitoring to assess diabetes development in cystic fibrosis patients. Endocrinology, Diabetes and Nutrition. 2018;**65**(1):45-51

[39] Ode KL et al. Oral glucose tolerance testing in children with cystic fibrosis. Pediatric Diabetes. 2010;**11**(7):487-492

[40] Scheuing N et al. Adherence to clinical care guidelines for cystic fibrosis-related diabetes in 659 German/Austrian patients. Journal of Cystic Fibrosis. 2014;**13**(6):730-736

[41] Annual Data Report 2018. UK Cystic Fibrosis Registry. 2019. Available from: https://www.cysticfibrosis.org.uk/the-work-we-do/uk-cf-registry/reporting-and-resources

[42] Grabert M, Schweiggert F, Holl RW. A framework for diabetes documentation and quality management in Germany: 10 years of experience with DPV. Computer Methods and Programs in Biomedicine. 2002;**69**(2):115-121

[43] Sawicki GS, Sellers DE, Robinson WM. High treatment burden in adults with cystic fibrosis: Challenges to disease self-management. Journal of Cystic Fibrosis. 2009;**8**(2):91-96

[44] Ziaian T et al. Treatment burden and health-related quality of life of children with diabetes, cystic fibrosis and asthma. Journal of Paediatrics and Child Health. 2006;**42**(10):596-600

[45] Scheuing N et al. Why is insulin pump treatment rarely used in adolescents and young adults with cystic fibrosis-related diabetes? Pediatric Diabetes. 2015;**16**(1):10-15

[46] Konrad K et al. Cystic fibrosis-related diabetes compared with type 1 and type 2 diabetes in adults. Diabetes/Metabolism Research and Reviews. 2013;**29**(7):568-575

[47] Rosenecker J et al. Diabetes mellitus and cystic fibrosis: Comparison of clinical parameters in patients treated with insulin versus oral glucose-lowering agents. Pediatric Pulmonology. 2001;**32**(5):351-355

[48] Rabe A, Disser J, Fromter E. Cl^- channel inhibition by glibenclamide is not specific for the CFTR-type Cl^- channel. Pflügers Archiv. 1995;**429**(5):659-662

[49] Schultz BD et al. Glibenclamide blockade of CFTR chloride channels. The American Journal of Physiology. 1996;**271**(2 Pt 1):L192-L200

[50] Sheppard DN, Robinson KA. Mechanism of glibenclamide inhibition of cystic fibrosis transmembrane conductance regulator Cl^- channels expressed in a murine cell line. The Journal of Physiology. 1997;**503**(Pt 2):333-346

[51] Cai Z, Lansdell KA, Sheppard DN. Inhibition of heterologously expressed cystic fibrosis transmembrane conductance regulator Cl^- channels by non-sulphonylurea hypoglycaemic agents. British Journal of Pharmacology. 1999;**128**(1):108-118

[52] Moran A, Phillips J, Milla C. Insulin and glucose excursion following premeal insulin lispro or repaglinide in cystic fibrosis-related diabetes. Diabetes Care. 2001;**24**(10):1706-1710

[53] Onady GM, Stolfi A. Insulin and oral agents for managing cystic fibrosis-related diabetes. Cochrane Database of Systematic Reviews. 2016;**4**:CD004730

[54] Moran A et al. Insulin therapy to improve BMI in cystic fibrosis-related

diabetes without fasting hyperglycemia results of the cystic fibrosis related diabetes therapy trial. Diabetes Care. 2009;**32**(10):1783-1788

[55] UK Cystic Fibrosis Trust Diabetes Working Group. Management of CF related diabetes—Report of the UK CF trust Diabetes working group(article online). 2004. Available from: http://www.cftrust.org.uk/aboutcf/publications/consensusdoc/diabetes.pdf

[56] Godbout A et al. No relationship between mean plasma glucose and glycated haemoglobin in patients with cystic fibrosis-related diabetes. Diabetes & Metabolism. 2008;**34**(6 Pt 1):568-573. Available from: https://doi.org/10.1016/j.jcf.2020.03.002

[57] Middleton PG et al. Australian standards of care for cystic fibrosis-related diabetes. Respirology. 2014;**19**(2):185-192

[58] Konrad K et al. Comparison of cystic fibrosis-related diabetes with type 1 diabetes based on a German/Austrian Pediatric Diabetes Registry. Diabetes Care. 2013;**36**(4):879-886

[59] Frost F et al. Continuous glucose monitoring guided insulin therapy is associated with improved clinical outcomes in cystic fibrosis-related diabetes. Journal of Cystic Fibrosis. 2018;**17**(6):798-803

[60] van den Berg JMW et al. Microvascular complications in patients with cystic fibrosis-related diabetes (CFRD). Journal of Cystic Fibrosis. 2008;**7**(6):515-519

[61] Schwarzenberg SJ et al. Microvascular complications in cystic fibrosis-related diabetes. Diabetes Care. 2007;**30**(5):1056-1061

[62] Roberts R et al. Retinal screening of patients with cystic fibrosis-related diabetes in Wales—A real eye opener. Journal of Cystic Fibrosis. 2015;**14**(2):282-284

[63] Eenkhoorn V et al. Diabetic keto-acidosis as a presentation of cystic fibrosis-related diabetes: A case report. Journal of Diabetes and its Complications. 2011;**25**(2):137-141

[64] Adler AI et al. Hyperglycemia and death in cystic fibrosis-related diabetes. Diabetes Care. 2011;**34**(7):1577-1578

[65] Haliloglu B et al. Hypoglycemia is common in children with cystic fibrosis and seen predominantly in females. Pediatric Diabetes. 2017;**18**(7):607-613

[66] Radike K et al. Prognostic relevance of hypoglycemia following an oral glucose challenge for cystic fibrosis-related diabetes. Diabetes Care. 2011;**34**(4):e43

[67] Ramsey BW et al. A CFTR potentiator in patients with cystic fibrosis and the G551D mutation. The New England Journal of Medicine. 2011;**365**(18):1663-1672

[68] Bellin MD et al. Insulin secretion improves in cystic fibrosis following ivacaftor correction of CFTR: A small pilot study. Pediatric Diabetes. 2013;**14**(6):417-421

[69] Kelly A et al. Islet hormone and incretin secretion in cystic fibrosis following 4-months of ivacaftor therapy. American Journal of Respiratory and Critical Care Medicine. 2018;**378**(12):1142

[70] Wainwright CE et al. Lumacaftor-ivacaftor in patients with cystic fibrosis homozygous for Phe508del CFTR. The New England Journal of Medicine. 2015;**373**(3):220-231

[71] Li A et al. Continuous glucose monitoring in youth with cystic fibrosis treated with lumacaftor-ivacaftor. Journal of Cystic Fibrosis. 2019;**18**(1):144-149

[72] Misgault B et al. Effect of one-year lumacaftor-ivacaftor treatment on glucose tolerance abnormalities in cystic fibrosis patients. Journal of Cystic Fibrosis. DOI: 10.1016/j.jcf.2020.03.002

[73] Scheuing N et al. High variability in oral glucose tolerance among 1,128 patients with cystic fibrosis: A multicenter screening study. PLoS One. 2014;**9**(11):e112578

[74] Middleton PG et al. Elexacaftor-tezacaftor-ivacaftor for cystic fibrosis with a single Phe508del allele. The New England Journal of Medicine. 2019;**381**(19):1809-1819

Chapter 3

Detection and Management of Early Glucose Abnormalities in Cystic Fibrosis

Katerina Theocharous, Bernadette Prentice, Charles F. Verge, Adam Jaffé and Shihab Hameed

Abstract

With advances in technology, it is now possible to detect the emergence of glucose abnormalities in cystic fibrosis with improved sensitivity, and from a very early age. These abnormalities are increasingly recognized as predictors of clinical decline, raising the possibility that early intervention may slow or prevent this deterioration. In this chapter, we will review the available literature on methods of detecting glucose abnormalities in cystic fibrosis (random and fasting glucose, HbA_{1c}, oral glucose tolerance testing, and continuous glucose monitoring), and detail their advantages and possible limitations in the interpretation of glycemic data. We will also discuss treatment outcomes of early intervention, prior to the diagnosis of diabetes as currently defined.

Keywords: cystic fibrosis-related diabetes, glucose, insulin, abnormal glucose tolerance, indeterminate glycaemia, impaired glucose tolerance, oral glucose tolerance test, continuous glucose monitoring

1. Introduction

Historically, cystic fibrosis (CF) caused fatal respiratory failure in early childhood [1, 2], but proactive multidisciplinary care has increased life expectancy to ~44 years [3]. With longer survival, co-morbidities have become more prevalent, the commonest being cystic fibrosis-related diabetes (CFRD) [4, 5]. This is associated with poorer clinical status [6–21], quality of life [22, 23], and life expectancy [16, 24, 25] relative to non-diabetic CF patients.

CFRD is distinct from other diabetes mellitus etiologies, including type 1 (T1D) and type 2 (T2D) (see **Table 1**) [4, 5]. It is caused primarily by chronic pancreatitis [26–30] with progressive insulin deficiency [9, 11, 31], particularly during first-phase insulin secretion [8, 9, 11, 19, 32–40]. Variations in peripheral insulin sensitivity also contribute to CFRD [20, 41]; hyperglycemia progressively induces insulin resistance via downregulation of glucose transporters [42–44], and insulin sensitivity decreases with inflammation, use of exogenous glucocorticoids, and puberty [45–49]. In CF, the depleted and dysfunctional pancreatic β-cells may be unable to compensate for this, producing early intermittent hyperglycemia progressing to fasting hyperglycemia [35, 44, 50].

IntechOpen

	Type 1 diabetes	Type 2 diabetes	CFRD
Prevalence	0.2%	11%	35% (likely underestimated due to lack of testing)
Onset	Usually acute	Insidious	Insidious
Peak age of onset	Childhood or adulthood	Adulthood	Ages 18–24
Usual body habitus	Normal	Overweight	Underweight, normal, or sometimes overweight (due to CF therapy success)
Likely pathophysiology	β-cell dysfunction & destruction, primarily autoimmune with genetic & possible environmental causes	Peripheral insulin resistance & subsequent β-cell stress	β-cell destruction due to inspissated pancreatic secretions, inflammation, and replacement with fibrosis & amyloid, plus a component of β-cell dysfunction
Insulin deficiency	Nearly complete	Partial and variable	Severe but not complete
Insulin resistance	Variable	Severe	Variable depending on circumstances (e.g. glycemic control, pubertal stage, use of glucocorticoids, inflammation)
Ketoacidosis risk	High	Low	Low
Pharmacological & dietary therapy	• Insulin • Dietary monitoring to ensure appropriate insulin dosage	• Insulin or oral anti-hypoglycemics • Low-calorie, low-carbohydrate, low-fat diet	• Insulin • Continuation of CF-specific diet, designed to prevent wasting: high-calorie, high-carbohydrate, high-fat
Complications	Microvascular & macrovascular disease	Microvascular & macrovascular disease	• Decline in nutritional status & lung function, associated with early mortality • Microvascular disease
Likeliest cause of death	Macrovascular disease	Macrovascular disease	CF pulmonary disease

Table 1.
Comparison of common etiologies of diabetes. Adapted from Moran et al. [4].

CFRD is usually preceded by a spectrum of abnormal glucose tolerance (AGT) on oral glucose tolerance testing (OGTT), including impaired fasting glucose (IFG), indeterminate glucose tolerance (INDET), and impaired glucose tolerance (IGT) [4, 51]. There may be 'waxing and waning' of glucose tolerance between these categories [19, 52–55], probably due to variations in insulin sensitivity [35, 44]. Nevertheless, large prospective cohort studies report overall deterioration in CF patients' glucose tolerance over life [16, 20, 53, 54, 56]. The date of onset of CFRD is considered to be the first time a patient meets diagnostic criteria, even if glucose abnormalities subsequently resolve due to improvement in insulin sensitivity [4]. This is because studies utilizing this definition report correlations between CFRD duration, microvascular disease prevalence [57], and mortality [16, 56].

Taken together, these factors explain why CFRD becomes more common with age. Prevalence is ~1.5% in CF patients aged <10 years, but ~15% in those aged 11–17 and ~50% in those aged ≥18 [8, 16, 58]. The American Diabetes Association (ADA) recommends annual screening from age 10, using 2-h OGTT [59]. CFRD can also be diagnosed using clinical status, random blood glucose, fasting plasma glucose, and glycated hemoglobin (HbA_{1c}) [4, 60, 61]. In clinically-stable outpatients with CF, diagnostic criteria are identical to those used for other etiologies of diabetes mellitus [4], and are shown in **Table 2**. Recently, continuous glucose monitoring (CGM) has also been used to investigate glucose abnormalities in CF patients. This method is not yet widely recommended for diagnosis of diabetes, but it is often used to monitor glycemic control or assist insulin dosage [62]. Moreover, CGM often detects even earlier CF-related glucose abnormalities than OGTT, in the form of intermittent postprandial glucose excursions [63].

This chapter compiles research on use of each glucose measurement method in CF patients, with special focus on pre-diabetic patients. The benefits and limitations of each method will be explored to help ascertain when their usage might be appropriate. In the process, we will examine correlations between early glucose abnormalities and clinical decline. Finally, we will review preliminary evidence of improved long-term outcomes with insulin treatment of early glucose abnormalities, supporting their detection and management in routine practice.

Glucose measurement method	Diagnostic criteria		
	Normal ranges	Pre-diabetic ranges	Diabetic ranges
Clinical status	Classical symptoms of hyperglycemia, including polyuria, polydipsia, and hyperglycemic crisis, may assist diagnosis of diabetes when combined with other positive diagnostic tests. Some CF-specific definitions also consider unexplained decline in lung function & nutritional status to be classical symptoms.		
HbA_{1c}	≤5.6% (38 mmol/mol)	5.7–6.4% (39–46 mmol/mol)	≥6.5% (48 mmol/mol)
Random blood glucose	—	—	≥11.1 mmol/L (200 mg/dL)
Fasting plasma glucose	<5.6 mmol/L (100 mg/dL)	**IFG:** ≥5.6 mmol/L (100 mg/dL), <7.0 mmol/L (126 mg/dL)	≥7.0 mmol/L (126 mg/dL)
2-h OGTT	*0 min:* <5.6 mmol/L (100 mg/dL) *2 h:* <7.8 mmol/L (140 mg/dL)	All categories constitute **AGT** **IFG:** *0 min:* ≥5.6 mmol/L (100 mg/dL), <7.0 mmol/L (126 mg/dL) *2 h:* N/A **INDET:** *0 min:* <7.0 mmol/L (126 mg/dL) *OGTT midpoints:* ≥11.1 mmol/L (200 mg/dL) *2 h:* <7.8 mmol/L (140 mg/dL) **IGT:** *0 min:* <7.0 mmol/L (126 mg/dL) *2 h:* ≥7.8 mmol/L (140 mg/dL), <11.1 mmol/L (200 mg/dL)	*0 min:* ≥7.0 mmol/L (126 mg/dL) *AND/OR* *2 h:* ≥11.1 mmol/L (200 mg/dL)
CGM	Usually <7.8 mmol/L (140 mg/dL)	Elevations ≥7.8 mmol/L (140 mg/dL) are referred to as **glucose excursions**, but there are no standardized criteria correlating them with AGT or diabetes.	

HbA_{1c} = glycated hemoglobin. OGTT = oral glucose tolerance testing. IFG = impaired fasting glucose. AGT = abnormal glucose tolerance. INDET = indeterminate glucose tolerance. IGT = impaired glucose tolerance. CGM = continuous glucose monitoring.

Table 2.
Diagnostic criteria of glucose measurement methods commonly used in CF. Diagnosis must occur during clinical stability, defined as no pulmonary exacerbations during the past 6 weeks and no current systemic glucocorticoids. It is also recommended that any positive fasting plasma glucose, HbA_{1c}, or OGTT is repeated at a later date. Non-CGM diagnostic criteria are from the American Diabetes Association [59, 64]. CGM diagnostic criteria are from the Juvenile Diabetes Research Foundation Continuous Glucose Monitoring Study Group [65].

2. Benefits and limitations of conventional methods used to diagnose glucose abnormalities in CF

2.1 Clinical status and/or random blood glucose

The ADA allows diagnosis of CFRD following one random blood glucose measurement ≥11.1 mmol/L, provided that it is combined with polyuria, polydipsia, or hyperglycemic crisis [59]. However, symptomatic hyperglycemia or hyperglycemic crisis is extremely rare in CFRD [4]. In Lanng et al.'s seminal 5-year prospective cohort study of 191 CF patients receiving annual OGTT, only 33% of those diagnosed with CFRD had polyuria or polydipsia [54]. Moreover, in a cross-sectional study of all 60 patients aged ≥10 years at a Brazilian CF center, age at diagnosis was significantly lower for patients diagnosed using OGTT as opposed to clinical criteria (13.5 years vs. 22.3 years), implying much earlier detection of disease [66].

Some centers compensate by accepting unexplained decline in lung function or nutritional status as classical symptoms of hyperglycemia (see Section 3) [67]. In one cross-sectional study of 91 CF patients not known to be diabetic, these modified clinical criteria detected OGTT-diagnosed CFRD with 58% sensitivity [68], which is an improvement over other studies but still suboptimal for a screening test.

2.2 HbA_{1c}

HbA_{1c}, i.e. glycated hemoglobin as a percentage of total hemoglobin, is commonly used to monitor glycemic control in diabetes mellitus. It usually reflects average blood glucose over the life of an erythrocyte (~3 months) [64, 69]. However, CF patients with CFRD, INDET or IGT rarely have a significantly-higher HbA_{1c} than those with normal glucose tolerance (NGT) [11, 70–73], and even statistically-significant differences tend to be of <1% magnitude [8, 34, 40, 74, 75]. Godbout et al.'s study of 13 CFRD patients also found that HbA_{1c} did not correlate with mean plasma glucose, as calculated using fingerprick self-monitoring [76].

Numerous hypotheses have been espoused to explain HbA_{1c}'s relatively poor correlation with glucose tolerance in CF. These include insufficient duration of transient CF-related post-prandial hyperglycemia, which is often limited to the early phase of insulin secretion; alteration of hemoglobin glycation by hypoxia; iron deficiency, which is a common comorbidity of CF; and increased erythrocyte turnover in the context of chronic inflammation [1, 4, 5, 76, 77]. This implies that HbA_{1c} may vary with degree of inflammation [78], and that *trends* in HbA_{1c} may be more useful for predicting deterioration in glucose tolerance. Supporting this, Lanng et al.'s 5-year prospective cohort study found significant differences in median HbA_{1c} between patients who consistently had NGT (5.2%), patients who varied between NGT and IGT (5.3%), patients who developed CFRD during the study (5.8%), and patients who entered the study with a diagnosis of CFRD (6.5%) [54].

It has also been hypothesized that poor correlation between mean plasma glucose and HbA_{1c} may be confounded by use of fingerprick tests to measure glucose, since these can easily miss CF-related hyperglycaemic peaks due to their relative infrequency [76]. In two studies of CF and CFRD patients, mean plasma glucose was estimated using 2–7 days of CGM rather than fingerprick self-monitoring, and strongly correlated with HbA_{1c} (r = 0.86–0.89) [75, 79].

These findings have regenerated interest in potentially using HbA_{1c} to screen for CF-related glucose abnormalities, especially because it is much more convenient than OGTT. However, computing HbA_{1c} thresholds suitable for CFRD screening has proved challenging. Some studies do report almost 100% sensitivity for OGTT-defined CFRD using HbA_{1c} thresholds of 6.0–7.5% [40, 80–82], but all have small sample sizes, and most either did not calculate sensitivity to CF-related AGT [81] or report low values, ~20–50% [80, 82]. Therefore, HbA_{1c} may not detect CFRD and its complications until late. Moreover, most evidence suggests that the diagnostic threshold for CFRD, HbA_{1c} ≥6.5%, has poor sensitivity compared to OGTT [54, 83–85].

Lowering the diagnostic threshold for HbA_{1c} abnormalities does increase sensitivity to both CFRD and AGT, but the thresholds required to achieve sufficient sensitivity for screening generally have unacceptably low specificity [60]. There is also wide variation in the sensitivities and specificities reported by different studies using the same HbA_{1c} threshold; this may be due to differences in type of HbA_{1c} assay [74, 86] and timing of the studies relative to the institution's routine OGTT screening [87]. Yung et al., conducting a cross-sectional study of 91 CF patients not known to be diabetic, but also not previously routinely screened, found that HbA_{1c} ≥6.1% had 83% sensitivity for OGTT-diagnosed CFRD [68]. However, more recent studies with similar designs report only 30–50% sensitivity [39, 82, 88, 89].

Given this uncertainty, the current advice from the ADA is that HbA_{1c} should not be used to screen for CF-related glucose abnormalities [59]. HbA_{1c} is still recommended for monitoring glycemic control in CFRD, although normal results must be interpreted with caution [4, 78]. It has also been suggested that HbA_{1c} might be a useful adjunct to OGTT in screening, as its results may fluctuate less and hence, may more accurately predict long-term risk of glucose abnormalities. In a recent 6-year retrospective cohort study of 50 NGT adults with CF followed up with annual OGTT, HbA_{1c} ≥5.6% had OR 3.49 for development of IGT or CFRD [90].

2.3 Fasting glucose

In 2003, the ADA briefly sanctioned fasting plasma glucose as an alternative to OGTT in CFRD screening, because there were insufficient data supporting insulin therapy for CFRD without fasting hyperglycemia [91]. However, subsequent studies have demonstrated similar insulin-induced clinical improvements in patients with and without fasting hyperglycemia [16, 92], and treatment of CFRD without fasting hyperglycemia is now standard practice [4]. Only 16–25% of patients diagnosed with CFRD on OGTT have fasting hyperglycemia [8, 54, 68, 81].

Use of fasting glucose to detect pre-diabetic stages on the glucose tolerance spectrum remains somewhat contentious in CF. Most studies report that fasting plasma glucose does not significantly differ between CF patients with NGT, INDET or IGT [39, 72, 93]. The ADA does use fasting glucose to define one pre-diabetic glucose tolerance category, IFG (5.6–6.9 mmol/L), and suggested in 2003 that screening OGTTs could be limited to IFG patients [94]. A prospective cohort study of 1128 CF patients aged 10–64 found that this approach would reduce number of OGTTs by 67%, but miss 17.8% of CFRD and IGT [94]. In a cross-sectional analysis of 73 children with CF, IFG had 100% sensitivity for CFRD, but only 25% sensitivity for IGT [11].

Finally, like HbA_{1c}, there is debate regarding the utility of IFG as an adjunctive test for predicting long-term risk of CFRD. Frohnert et al. found no significant relationship [95], but Schmid et al. found that IFG generated OR 2.72 for CFRD [96].

2.4 Oral glucose tolerance testing

As discussed above, other conventional diagnostic tests have <100% sensitivity for CFRD compared to OGTT. Therefore, OGTT remains the recommended screening test in CF. It is also the only test with standardized definitions of multiple pre-diabetic glucose abnormalities, all demonstrated to predict development of CFRD [96].

Nevertheless, there are several issues with the 2-h OGTT. It may be more inconvenient and resource-intensive than other glucose measurement methods, which is of particular concern in CF because patients and clinics already face a high treatment burden from other aspects of CF care [97]. It also requires patient co-operation, which can be difficult when assessing children [93]. Patients are expected to consume at least 150 g (600 kcal) of carbohydrates for 3 days before an OGTT, then fast for 8 h overnight and be tested early the next morning [59]. They must drink a solution containing a 1.75 g/kg glucose load, preferably within 5 min, then lie or sit quietly for 2 h [64]. In a standard OGTT, venous blood is sampled twice: immediately before ingestion of the load, and at 120 min (BG_{120}). Many CF centers also take hourly or 30-minutely samples to detect post-prandial hyperglycemia that resolves before 2 h [59]. As described earlier, these transient post-prandial glucose excursions are very common in CF, due to selective impairment of early insulin secretion. Our group previously performed OGTT with 30-minutely sampling in 33 children with CF aged 10–19, and found that peak venous insulin concentration was delayed until 90–120 min, producing an early venous glucose peak at 60–90 min [9] (**Figure 1**).

The inconvenience of OGTT may contribute to poor patient uptake of CFRD screening [98–100]. In 2018, the Cystic Fibrosis Foundation Patient Registry reported that the average CF center was screening just 61.3% of adolescents and 32.8% of adults [100]. Rates of utilization of other glucose measurement methods, such as HbA_{1c} and fasting glucose, were much higher (92.3% for adolescents and 89.6% for adults), suggesting that the main barrier to screening is the OGTT itself [100]. Suggested solutions include shortening the OGTT to 60 or 90 min [83] or replacing it with the 50-g non-fasting 1-h glucose challenge test [89, 101], which is currently used to screen for gestational diabetes mellitus in healthy women [101]. These modified OGTT protocols are not standard recommended practice [4].

There are also other issues with the OGTT that likely cannot be resolved by simply shortening it. Its diagnostic thresholds are not specific to CF and may be insensitive to CF-related clinical decline (see Section 3). OGTT results also frequently fluctuate in CF, with a large multicenter prospective cohort study finding a variability coefficient 1.5–1.8 times higher than in the general population [55]. Similarly, in two 4–5 year prospective cohort studies, 18–58% of AGT patients demonstrated overall improvement in glucose tolerance category, while only 14–22% demonstrated deterioration [19, 54].

Finally, even with venous sampling at additional timepoints, the peak blood glucose measurements recorded during OGTT may poorly reflect peak blood glucose achieved by CF patients in daily life [4, 60, 61]. After all, the OGTT's 1.75 g/kg load contains less glucose than most CF patients' everyday meals [61, 98]. This has prompted research into CF-related glucose abnormalities using CGM, a technology that can screen for glucose excursions over a longer interval of everyday life and high calorie CF diet.

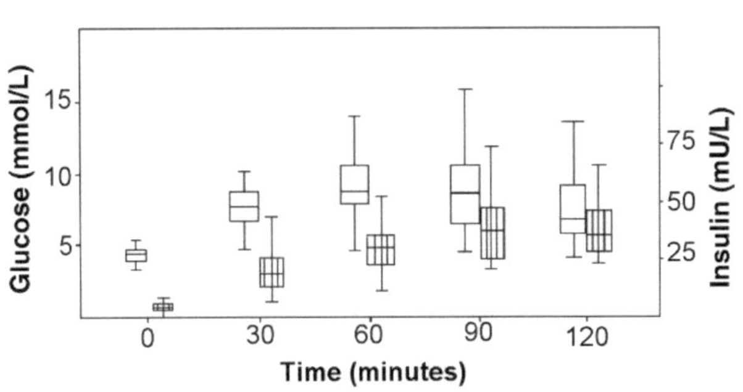

Figure 1.
Venous blood glucose (□) and insulin (▦) in 30-minutely samples over a 2-h oral glucose tolerance test, as measured in 33 children with CF aged 10–19. Boxes indicate interquartile range, horizontal lines indicate median, whiskers indicate 5th and 95th percentiles. Figure taken from Hameed et al. [9].

2.5 Continuous glucose monitoring

Most CGM systems consist of two parts: a sterile sensor, worn subcutaneously for up to 14 days, and a transmitter attached to the sensor that measures interstitial fluid glucose every 30 s, recording an average every 5 min [97] (**Figure 2**). Some systems do not require a separate sensor, instead measuring interstitial fluid glucose via an electrical current applied across intact skin, but issues have been reported with skin reactions and inaccuracy [102]. Interstitial fluid glucose reflects capillary glucose with a 4–20 min delay [103].

CGM has been validated against OGTT in children with CF of all glucose tolerance categories [104] and non-diabetic adolescents and adults with CF [105]. A subsequent study of this latter group found that they differed significantly from healthy controls in mean CGM glucose (+14.1%) and presence of CGM peaks ≥11.1 mmol/L (+33%), but not in the conventional diagnostic measures of fasting glucose, BG_{120}, and HbA_{1c} [106]. Moreover, 70% of CF patients undertaking simultaneous CGM and OGTT had their CGM peak *outside* OGTT [106]. This was the beginning of a substantial body of evidence demonstrating the superior sensitivity of CGM to CF-related glucose excursions above OGTT diagnostic thresholds, with numerous studies finding CGM glucose peaks ≥7.8 or 11.1 mmol/L in 71–93% of patients classified as NGT on recent OGTT [14, 31, 85, 98, 107, 108]. In a 5-year prospective cohort study of 21 adults with CF, 83% had their CGM peak and BG_{120} fall in different diagnostic categories, and for 93% the CGM-identified category was worse. Again, this suggests the superior sensitivity of CGM over OGTT [98].

Most of this evidence, particularly in children, is limited by small sample sizes [14, 85, 98, 107, 108] and lack of non-CF controls [14, 85, 98, 108]. However, it is logical that the increased duration and frequency of glucose monitoring facilitated by CGM, and the opportunity to incorporate the patient's usual diet and physical activity, facilitates more sensitive detection of glucose excursions [109]. CGM is also generally easier and better tolerated than OGTT [78]. While sensors and transmitters are expensive, and staff do require training on their usage, they have become more user-friendly, smaller and cheaper over time [73, 110]. The newest devices can be inserted rapidly during a clinic appointment, do not require calibration against fingerpricks, and can be removed by patients or carers without medical supervision [97].

CGM does have one major disadvantage compared to OGTT. The clinical significance of the mild glucose excursions that it detects are still being determined; consequently, there is no standardized system for recognizing and describing clinically relevant CGM findings, and no universally accepted threshold for initiation

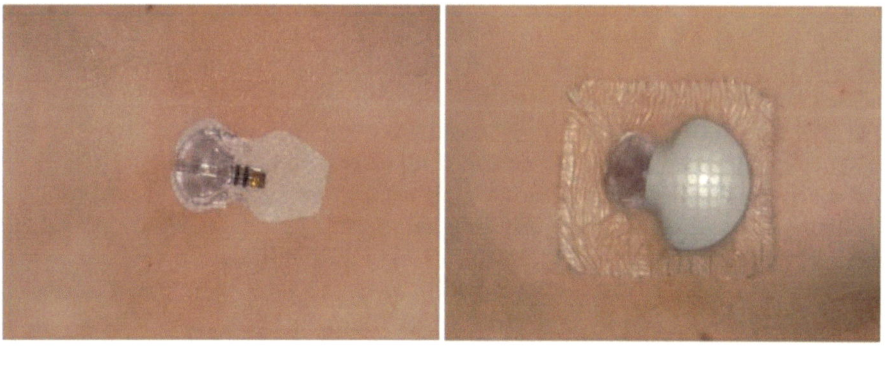

Figure 2.
Continuous glucose monitor sensor, before and after attachment of the transmitter. 'CGM set' and 'Continuous Glucose Monitor' by Sara Bassett are licensed under CC BY-NC-SA 2.0.

of treatment [97]. Common variables computed by CGM software include average sensor glucose, maximum glucose, area under the curve of glucose per day ($AUC_{glucose}$/day), percentage time spent above thresholds (e.g. 7.8 or 11.1 mmol/L), number of excursions ≥11.1 mmol/L, and measures of glycemic variability, such as standard deviation of average sensor glucose [103]. All these parameters have been correlated with HbA_{1c} in CF patients [75], and many have been correlated with clinical outcomes. However, these studies report heterogeneous findings and rarely include substantial prospective follow-up (see Section 3) [84].

Given all these factors, CGM is not yet widely recommended for CFRD diagnosis or screening [4]. However, it is used in some centers for diagnosis and screening, follow-up of borderline diagnostic tests, and investigation of patients who cannot or refuse to undergo OGTT [31, 111, 112]. Like HbA_{1c}, it may also be useful as an adjunctive test for predicting long-term risk of CF-related glucose abnormalities. In a prospective cohort study of 17 children with CF, all those who had glucose excursions ≥11.1 mmol/L on CGM developed either CFRD or IGT with INDET over a period of 2.5 years, irrespective of their glucose tolerance at baseline [107].

3. Clinical significance of early glucose abnormalities in CF, as detected using various glucose measurement techniques

3.1 Defining clinically significant sequelae of CFRD: the importance of lung function & nutritional status

CFRD is well-understood to have a differing profile of sequelae as compared to T1D or T2D. Macrovascular disease is uncommon outside of case reports [1, 4, 5, 113], and although screening for microvascular disease should be routinely undertaken [59], microvascular complications are uncommon until at least 5–10 years of CFRD with fasting hyperglycemia [57, 114, 115]. Therefore they are substantially predated by declines in lung function [6–21, 116–118] and nutritional status [7, 9–12, 14, 117], both of which are significant predictors of early mortality in CF [10, 11, 16, 18, 25, 56, 119]. Four large cohort studies also report higher annual frequency in diabetic vs. non-diabetic CF patients of pulmonary exacerbations requiring intravenous antibiotics or hospitalization [10, 21, 39, 120], and it was recently demonstrated that diabetic CF patients have reduced recovery of baseline forced expiratory volume in 1 sec as a percentage of predicted (FEV_1%) following pulmonary exacerbations [116].

A causative relationship between CFRD, impaired lung function, and poor nutritional status is implied by the clinical improvements seen following insulin therapy [13, 92, 120–122], and is also biologically plausible on several accounts. Insulin is a powerfully anabolic hormone, therefore insulin deficiency combined with CF's increased metabolic requirements promotes catabolism with nutritional decline [9, 93, 123, 124]. Regarding lung function and pulmonary exacerbations, hyperglycemia is known to promote respiratory tract infections (RTIs) both systemically, via pro-inflammatory and immunosuppressive effects [125, 126], and locally, via glucose leakage into airway secretions, which could promote pathogen growth [125, 127–130]. Several cohort studies report higher prevalence in diabetic vs. non-diabetic CF patients of certain RTIs, including *Pseudomonas aeruginosa* [10, 19, 117, 131], *Staphylococcus aureus* [132, 133], and *Burkholderia cepacia* [10, 117, 132].

Finally, hyperglycemia can also impair lung function through non-infective pathways. It has been associated with restrictive lung disease in T1D and T2D (via non-enzymatic glycation of collagen and elastin) [134], and with inflammatory and proteolytic lung destruction in CFRD [135–137]. Lung proteolysis may be exacerbated by protein catabolism [19, 122], which can furthermore weaken respiratory muscles [138, 139] and impair immunoprotein synthesis during RTIs [61]. This may explain why lung function in CF also correlates with nutritional status [6, 7, 140–142].

3.2 Decline in clinical status prior to diagnosis of CFRD

Numerous cohort and case-control studies examining the 1–5 years before CFRD diagnosis report decline in lung function [19, 35, 38, 92, 143–146] and nutritional status [19, 35, 38, 92, 143, 144] in pre-diabetic patients, or significantly reduced values compared to non-diabetic CF controls [12, 17]. This suggests that pre-diabetic glucose abnormalities are clinically significant. Two case-control studies focusing specifically on pediatric populations also report that pre-diabetic children with CF have significantly lower height and weight velocities than non-diabetic CF controls [145, 146], with one study demonstrating differences up to 11 years before CFRD diagnosis [146]. These differing velocities produce steadily-widening gaps in height-for-age and weight-for-age, reaching statistically-significant sizes after CFRD diagnosis, usually around ages 15–19 [18, 146]. Importantly, this growing disparity seems to occur even if aggressive insulin therapy is commenced at diagnosis [144], and although it may narrow with prolonged therapy, it may not fully correct [18, 144, 147]. Therefore, optimizing clinical outcomes in CFRD may require treatment of pre-diabetic abnormalities, highlighting the importance of glucose measurement systems that can sensitively predict clinical decline.

3.3 Clinically significant pre-diabetic markers detectable using OGTT

Traditional OGTT diagnostic thresholds are not specific to CF – in fact, they were originally designed to predict T2D-associated microvascular disease in Pima Native Americans [148]. This may explain their apparent insensitivity to CF clinical outcomes. A few studies do report poorer lung function or nutritional status in IGT vs. NGT CF patients [37, 72], and several more identify IGT as a significant risk factor for substantial decline in $FEV_1\%$ over 4–5 years [19, 149]. However, most studies attempting to correlate IGT with contemporary lung function and nutritional status find no significant relationship [19, 33, 34, 39, 53, 70–73, 150–152].

A more successful non-conventional OGTT parameter is the additional glucose tolerance category of INDET, defined as blood glucose ≥11.1 mmol/L at an OGTT midpoint – most commonly 60 min (BG_{60}) – as opposed to 0 or 120 min [4]. BG_{60} has been shown to inversely correlate with BMI in children with CF, and correlates with $FEV_1\%$ and forced vital capacity as a percentage of predicted (FVC%) in both children [7] and adults [150]. In a subsequent study, INDET patients had mean $FEV_1\%$ comparable to CFRD patients, representing a significant reduction compared to NGT and IGT patients [71]. INDET has also been confirmed to predict development of CFRD (OR 2.81 over ~3.5 years) [93, 96].

Other OGTT parameters shown to predict $FEV_1\%$ in non-diabetic CF patients include higher peak glucose (BG_{max}) [9, 33, 72, 153], higher $AUC_{glucose}$ [124, 153], and reduced insulin secretion [34, 35, 72, 124]. Finally, a few studies have correlated $FEV_1\%$ with trajectories of deterioration in glucose tolerance [41, 154]. One prospective cohort study recruited 152 non-diabetic CF patients, and stratified them according to whether their glucose tolerance on OGTT improved, deteriorated or remained stable over 2 years [41]. While all patients experienced a decline in $FEV_1\%$, the extent of decline only reached statistical significance in patients of stable or deteriorating glucose tolerance, and those of deteriorating glucose tolerance also had a much larger drop than those of stable glucose tolerance (−6.1% vs. −1.6%) [41].

It is rarer for studies to report correlations between OGTT parameters and nutritional status [33–35, 41, 71, 72, 154], possibly because intensive dietician management of CF mitigates nutritional decline [133, 154]. Nevertheless, one seminal prospective cohort study inversely correlated age-adjusted height and BMI with $AUC_{glucose}$ [8], and a recent cross-sectional study found that lower-than-median insulin secretion at 60 min is independently associated with worse BMI [150]. In children, BMI (calculated as weight in kg divided by the square of height in meters) may be a less sensitive measure of nutritional status than weight-for-age, as poor linear growth may mask decline [146]. Nevertheless, Wooldridge et al. report a direct correlation between $AUC_{insulin}$ and BMI z-score in 146 NGT children with CF aged 5–20 [123], and our group has found that $AUC_{glucose}$ inversely correlates with age-adjusted weight, height and BMI in children aged ≤10 years [153]. Furthermore, in an earlier cohort study of 33 children aged 10–19, we found that higher BG_{max} was associated with decline in weight z-score, FEV_1% and FVC% over the past 12 months, and BG_{max} ≥8.2 mmol/L had 87% sensitivity and 70% specificity for a clinically significant decline in weight z-score [9]. By contrast, BG_{120} was no better than chance at detecting decline in weight z-score, and the conventional diagnostic threshold of 11.1 mmol/L had only 10% sensitivity [9]. These findings led us to propose an alternative system for classifying CF-related glucose abnormalities on OGTT, the Cystic Fibrosis Insulin Deficiency (CFID) stages (**Table 3**) [9].

3.4 Clinically significant pre-diabetic markers detectable using CGM

Six main studies have explored the clinical significance of CGM-based measures of CF-related early glucose abnormalities [9, 98, 111, 152, 155, 156]. Their results are compelling but heterogeneous. Taylor-Cousar et al. conducted a 5-year prospective cohort study of 17 originally non-diabetic CF patients, 7 of whom developed CFRD during observation [98]. In this subgroup, there was significant inverse correlation between peak glucose and BMI, and a trend towards correlation with FEV_1% [98]. Leclercq et al. also examined peak glucose, stratifying 38 NGT CF patients according to whether they had any peaks ≥11.1 mmol/L during 72-h CGM [155]. In the 'yes' group, there was significantly lower FEV_1% and FVC%, and increased risk of colonization with *P. aeruginosa* [155].

In the aforementioned study undertaken by our research group in 33 children with CF aged 10–19, we also showed that percentage time ≥7.8 mmol/L on CGM predicted 12-month rate of decline in weight z-score, FVC%, and FEV_1%. Similarly, on receiver operator characteristic (ROC) analysis, ≥4.5% time at ≥7.8 mmol/L on CGM was a sensitive and specific predictor of clinically significant decline in weight z-score and FVC% [9]. Frost et al. subsequently used these parameters to interpret the CGM results of 59 adults being investigated for CF-related glucose abnormalities [112]. They found that percentage time ≥7.8 mmol/L on CGM correlated with baseline FEV_1% and 12-month rate of decline [112].

In Chan et al.'s study of 88 children with CF aged 10–18, 12-month decline in FEV_1% and FVC% was predicted by multiple other CGM parameters: peak glucose, number of daily glucose excursions >11.1 mmol/L, mean amplitude of glycemic

Diagnostic category	0-min OGTT glucose	Max OGTT glucose	2-h OGTT glucose
CFID1	<7.0 mmol/L	≥8.2 mmol/L	<11.1 mmol/L
CFID2	<7.0 mmol/L	≥11.1 mmol/L	<11.1 mmol/L
CFID3	<7.0 mmol/L	*N/A*	≥11.1 mmol/L
CFID4	≥7.0 mmol/L	*N/A*	*N/A*

Table 3.
Cystic fibrosis insulin deficiency (CFID) classification system of CF-related glucose abnormalities, as proposed by Hameed et al. [9].

excursions, and standard deviation [152]. Brugha et al. investigated another glycemic variability measure, glucose interquartile ranges, in a 7-year retrospective cohort study [111]. On ROC analysis, ranges >1.95 mmol/L predicted CFRD with 60% sensitivity and 98% specificity, but did not correlate with BMI or FEV_1% [111].

Finally, our group recently conducted a cross-sectional study of 18 children with CF aged ≤5 years [156]. Even in this very young group, history of *P. aeruginosa* was predicted by mean glucose and percentage time at ≥7.8 mmol/L, and levels of inflammatory markers in bronchoalveolar lavage fluid were predicted by peak glucose, mean glucose, percentage time at ≥7.8 mmol/L, and standard deviation [156].

3.5 Clinically significant pre-diabetic markers detectable using other glucose measurement techniques

3.5.1 HbA_{1c} and alternative glycated proteins

Three studies report a weak inverse correlation between HbA_{1c} and lung function in non-diabetic CF patients ($r = -0.25$–0.3) [72, 73, 88], and one of these also found a direct correlation with number of infective pulmonary exacerbations per year [73]. In two more studies, $HbA_{1c} \geq 5.5$–5.8% predicted poorer FVC% [74] or FEV_1% [82]. Therefore HbA_{1c}, despite its insensitivity to CF-related glucose abnormalities, may be a useful harbinger of clinical decline when elevated.

Several studies have also investigated fructosamine, glycated albumin, and 1,5-anhydroglucitol as alternatives to HbA_{1c} in CF. These biomarkers are not dependent on the lifespan of erythrocytes, and have been shown to correlate with mean plasma glucose in CF as estimated using CGM [75]. However, evidence of their ability to predict glucose abnormalities and clinical decline in CF is currently mixed [11, 74, 157]. In one study, fractional serum fructosamine (FSF) ≥3.70 μmol/g predicted IGT and CFRD with 100% sensitivity and 67% specificity, and patients with elevated FSF also had significantly lower median FEV_1% (47% vs. 90%) [157].

3.5.2 Fasting glucose

Early evidence suggests that fasting glucose, including IFG, does not correlate with clinical status in CF [53, 95]. In one case-control study, IFG actually predicted *better* lung function than normal fasting glucose in some patient subgroups, particularly children with simultaneous IGT [95]. It was hypothesized that IFG may represent a physiological adaptation to CF, with hepatic glucose production upregulated to meet increased baseline metabolic requirements [95].

4. Detection protocols for early glucose abnormalities and CFRD at the Sydney Children's Hospital, Randwick

Our institute, the Sydney Children's Hospital, provides one example of integrating multiple glucose measurement methods into routine practice. Children with CF are screened annually for glucose abnormalities from age 10, using OGTT with 30-minutely sampling. CGM is used to follow up borderline OGTTs, or to investigate children with clinically-suspected glucose abnormalities who have normal OGTTs or are unable to undergo OGTT. CGM excursions ≥11.1 mmol/L over 72 h of monitoring are considered severe abnormalities that warrant further investigation for possible insulin therapy. Moreover, some pre-diabetic children on OGTT are randomized to insulin therapy via the CF-IDEA trial (ClinicalTrials.gov Identifier NCT01100892, see Section 5).

5. Management of early glucose abnormalities in CF

Ultimately, the most clinically relevant measures of CF-related early glucose abnormalities are those that alter patient management. Therefore the long-term effects of actively treating early abnormalities is an important research question. Most studies have focused on insulin therapy, as insulin is currently the only recommended pharmacotherapy for CFRD (in part because of its anabolic effects) [59]. Emerging research has also explored oral anti-hypoglycemics [158], incretin modifiers [159], and CFTR modulators [160, 161].

It is already known that earlier diagnosis and treatment of CFRD, via OGTT screening programs, improves life expectancy and resolves historical sex differences in clinical outcomes (females with CFRD previously did worse than males) [16, 24]. Seven studies were identified trialing insulin therapy for CF patients who were pre-diabetic on OGTT [92, 122, 143, 162–164]. Five report statistically-significant improvements in lung function [122, 163, 165], nutritional status [122, 143, 164, 165], or rate of decline in either variable [163, 164], either intra-individually or relative to untreated controls. Moreover, five out of six studies assessing tolerability found no significantly-increased incidence of symptomatic hypoglycemia [92, 122, 143, 162, 164, 165]. Finally, one additional study has assessed the efficacy of insulin therapy initiated based on CGM, via retrospective analysis of all non-diabetic adults at a British CF center who had a CGM ordered between 2013 and 2016 [112]. Insulin was initiated if patients spent >4.5% time at >7.8 mmol/L on CGM, and if they recorded no clear triggers for these glucose excursions in a contemporary food diary. Patients treated with insulin demonstrated statistically-significant improvements in FEV_1% and weight within 3 months of treatment, and maintained an improvement in weight and annual rate of lung function decline at 12 months [112].

All this suggests that treatment of CF-related AGT may be beneficial. However, results are difficult to generalize, due to heterogeneity in studies' inclusions criteria, types of controls, and insulin regimens [166]. Studies are also limited by small sample sizes [92, 112, 122, 143, 162–165], short durations [92, 112, 122, 143, 162, 165], and mixed analysis of pre-diabetic and diabetic patients [92, 122], highlighting the need for large long-term randomized control trials. One such trial, CF-IDEA (ClinicalTrials.gov Identifier NCT01100892), is nearing completion. To date, CF-IDEA has recruited 86 participants aged ≥5 years at 5 participating sites, all non-diabetic on OGTT with BG_{max} 8.2 mmol/L to <11.1 mmol/L (CFID1) or ≥ 11.1 mmol/L (CFID2). Participants are randomized to observation only or to a once-daily insulin detemir (Levemir) for 12 months, with starting dose 0.1 units/kg/day, blood glucose self-monitoring intensively for 10 days and twice daily thereafter, and a blood glucose target range of 4–8 mmol/L. The main outcome factors are change in weight SDS, change in lung function, and frequency of hospitalization.

6. Conclusions

As patients with CF live longer, CFRD becomes an increasingly prevalent serious co-morbidity, associated with significant decline in lung function and nutritional status. Evidence suggests that this decline may begin years earlier, in the pre-diabetic phase. Currently, OGTT is the most sensitive licensed diagnostic tool for identifying pre-diabetic CF-related glucose abnormalities, but its utility is limited by inconvenience, high variability of results, and insensitivity of traditional diagnostic categories to CF-related glucose excursions and clinical decline.

Development of standardized interpretation systems for CGM may revolutionize detection of clinically relevant early glucose abnormalities. Results of randomized controlled trials of insulin treatment prior to onset of CFRD may alter the point at which insulin is offered.

Acknowledgements

SH, AJ and CFV have received funding from the National Health and Medical Research Council of Australia, Australasian Cystic Fibrosis Research Trust, Regional Diabetes Support Scheme, Sydney Children's Hospital Foundation, and Australasian Pediatric Endocrine Care Grant from Pfizer, and industry support from Novo Nordisk, Medtronic, and Abbott Diagnostics. BP has been awarded a fellowship from the Thoracic Society of Australia and New Zealand and Vertex, and a postgraduate scholarship from the National Health and Medical Research Council of Australia.

Author details

Katerina Theocharous[1], Bernadette Prentice[1,2], Charles F. Verge[1,3], Adam Jaffé[1,2] and Shihab Hameed[1,3,4]*

1 School of Women's and Children's Health, Faculty of Medicine, The University of New South Wales, Sydney, NSW, Australia

2 Department of Respiratory Medicine, Sydney Children's Hospital, Randwick, NSW, Australia

3 Department of Endocrinology, Sydney Children's Hospital, Randwick, NSW, Australia

4 Faculty of Medicine, University of Sydney, Sydney, NSW, Australia

*Address all correspondence to: s.hameed@unsw.edu.au

References

[1] Bridges N, Rowe R, Holt RIG. Unique challenges of cystic fibrosis-related diabetes. Diabetic Medicine. 2018;**35**(9):1181-1188

[2] Reid DW, Blizzard CL, Shugg DM, Flowers C, Cash C, Greville HM. Changes in cystic fibrosis mortality in Australia, 1979-2005. The Medical Journal of Australia. 2011;**195**(7):392-395

[3] Keogh RH, Szczesniak R, Taylor-Robinson D, Bilton D. Up-to-date and projected estimates of survival for people with cystic fibrosis using baseline characteristics: A longitudinal study using UK patient registry data. Journal of Cystic Fibrosis. 2018;**17**(2):218-227

[4] Moran A, Pillay K, Becker D, Granados A, Hameed S, Acerini CL. ISPAD clinical practice consensus guidelines 2018: Management of cystic fibrosis-related diabetes in children and adolescents. Pediatric Diabetes. 2018;**19**:64-74

[5] Kayani K, Mohammed R, Mohiaddin H. Cystic fibrosis-related diabetes. Frontiers in Endocrinology. 2018;**9**:20

[6] Kerem E, Viviani L, Zolin A, MacNeill S, Hatziagorou E, Ellemunter H, et al. Factors associated with FEV1 decline in cystic fibrosis: Analysis of the ECFS patient registry. The European Respiratory Journal. 2014;**43**(1):125-133

[7] Brodsky J, Dougherty S, Makani R, Rubenstein RC, Kelly A. Elevation of 1-hour plasma glucose during oral glucose tolerance testing is associated with worse pulmonary function in cystic fibrosis. Diabetes Care. 2011;**34**(2):292-295

[8] Bismuth E, Laborde K, Taupin P, Velho G, Ribault V, Jennane F, et al. Glucose tolerance and insulin secretion, morbidity, and death in patients with cystic fibrosis. The Journal of Pediatrics. 2008;**152**(4):540-545

[9] Hameed S, Morton JR, Jaffé A, Field PI, Belessis Y, Yoong T, et al. Early glucose abnormalities in cystic fibrosis are preceded by poor weight gain. Diabetes Care. 2010;**33**(2):221-226

[10] Marshall BC, Butler SM, Stoddard M, Moran AM, Liou TG, Morgan WJ, et al. Epidemiology of cystic fibrosis-related diabetes. The Journal of Pediatrics. 2005;**146**(5):681-687

[11] Elder DA, Wooldridge JL, Dolan LM, D'Alessio DA. Glucose tolerance, insulin secretion, and insulin sensitivity in children and adolescents with cystic fibrosis and no prior history of diabetes. The Journal of Pediatrics. 2007;**151**(6):653-658

[12] Lanng S, Thorsteinsson B, Nerup J, Koch C. Influence of the development of diabetes mellitus on clinical status in patients with cystic fibrosis. European Journal of Pediatrics. 1992;**151**(9):684-687

[13] Lanng S, Thorsteinsson B, Nerup J, Koch C. Diabetes mellitus in cystic fibrosis: Effect of insulin therapy on lung function and infections. Acta Paediatrica. 1994;**83**(8):849-853

[14] Moreau F, Weiller MA, Rosner V, Weiss L, Hasselmann M, Pinget M, et al. Continuous glucose monitoring in cystic fibrosis patients according to the glucose tolerance. Hormone and Metabolic Research. 2008;**40**(7):502-506

[15] Suratwala D, Chan JS, Kelly A, Meltzer LJ, Gallagher PR, Traylor J, et al. Nocturnal saturation and glucose tolerance in children with cystic fibrosis. Thorax. 2011;**66**(7):574-578

[16] Moran A, Dunitz J, Nathan B, Saeed A, Holme B, Thomas W. Cystic fibrosis-related diabetes: Current trends in prevalence, incidence, and mortality. Diabetes Care. 2009;**32**(9):1626-1631

[17] Rolon MA, Benali K, Munck A, Navarro J, Clement A, Tubiana-Rufi N, et al. Cystic fibrosis-related diabetes mellitus: Clinical impact of prediabetes and effects of insulin therapy. Acta Paediatrica. 2001;**90**(8):860-867

[18] Koch C, Rainisio M, Madessani U, Harms HK, Hodson ME, Mastella G, et al. Presence of cystic fibrosis-related diabetes mellitus is tightly linked to poor lung function in patients with cystic fibrosis: Data from the European epidemiologic registry of cystic fibrosis. Pediatric Pulmonology. 2001;**32**(5):343-350

[19] Milla CE, Warwick WJ, Moran A. Trends in pulmonary function in patients with cystic fibrosis correlate with the degree of glucose intolerance at baseline. American Journal of Respiratory and Critical Care Medicine. 2000;**162**(3 Pt 1):891-895

[20] Lombardo F, De Luca F, Rosano M, Sferlazzas C, Lucanto C, Arrigo T, et al. Natural history of glucose tolerance, beta-cell function and peripheral insulin sensitivity in cystic fibrosis patients with fasting euglycemia. European Journal of Endocrinology. 2003;**149**(1):53-59

[21] Limoli DH, Yang J, Khansaheb MK, Helfman B, Peng L, Stecenko AA, et al. Staphylococcus aureus and Pseudomonas aeruginosa co-infection is associated with cystic fibrosis-related diabetes and poor clinical outcomes. European Journal of Clinical Microbiology & Infectious Diseases. 2016;**35**(6):947-953

[22] Abbott J, Morton AM, Hurley MA, Conway SP. Longitudinal impact of demographic and clinical variables on health-related quality of life in cystic fibrosis. BMJ Open. 2015;**5**(5):e007418

[23] Kwong E, Desai S, Chong L, Lee K, Zheng J, Wilcox PG, et al. The impact of cystic fibrosis-related diabetes on health-related quality of life. Journal of Cystic Fibrosis. 2019;**18**(5):734-736

[24] Lewis C, Blackman SM, Nelson A, Oberdorfer E, Wells D, Dunitz J, et al. Diabetes-related mortality in adults with cystic fibrosis: Role of genotype and sex. American Journal of Respiratory and Critical Care Medicine. 2015;**191**(2):194-200

[25] Chamnan P, Shine BS, Haworth CS, Bilton D, Adler AI. Diabetes as a determinant of mortality in cystic fibrosis. Diabetes Care. 2010;**33**(2):311-316

[26] Bogdani M, Blackman SM, Ridaura C, Bellocq JP, Powers AC, Aguilar-Bryan L. Structural abnormalities in islets from very young children with cystic fibrosis may contribute to cystic fibrosis-related diabetes. Scientific Reports. 2017;**7**(1):17231

[27] Hart NJ, Aramandla R, Poffenberger G, Fayolle C, Thames AH, Bautista A, et al. Cystic fibrosis-related diabetes is caused by islet loss and inflammation. JCI Insight. 2018;**3**(8):e98240

[28] Iannucci A, Mukai K, Johnson D, Burke B. Endocrine pancreas in cystic fibrosis: An immunohistochemical study. Human Pathology. 1984;**15**(3):278-284

[29] Couce M, O'Brien TD, Moran A, Roche PC, Butler PC. Diabetes mellitus in cystic fibrosis is characterized by islet amyloidosis. The Journal of Clinical Endocrinology and Metabolism. 1996;**81**(3):1267-1272

[30] Löhr M, Goertchen P, Nizze H, Gould NS, Gould VE, Oberholzer M,

et al. Cystic fibrosis associated islet changes may provide a basis for diabetes: An immunocytochemical and morphometrical study. Virchows Archiv. A, Pathological Anatomy and Histopathology. 1989;**414**(2):179-185

[31] Mainguy C, Bellon G, Delaup V, Ginoux T, Kassai-Koupai B, Mazur S, et al. Sensitivity and specificity of different methods for cystic fibrosis-related diabetes screening: Is the oral glucose tolerance test still the standard? Journal of Pediatric Endocrinology & Metabolism. 2017;**30**(1):27-35

[32] Yung B, Noormohamed FH, Kemp M, Hooper J, Lant AF, Hodson ME. Cystic fibrosis-related diabetes: The role of peripheral insulin resistance and beta-cell dysfunction. Diabetic Medicine. 2002;**19**(3):221-226

[33] Anzeneder L, Kircher F, Feghelm N, Fischer R, Seissler J. Kinetics of insulin secretion and glucose intolerance in adult patients with cystic fibrosis. Hormone and Metabolic Research. 2011;**43**(5):355-360

[34] Costa M, Potvin S, Hammana I, Malet A, Berthiaume Y, Jeanneret A, et al. Increased glucose excursion in cystic fibrosis and its association with a worse clinical status. Journal of Cystic Fibrosis. 2007;**6**(6):376-383

[35] Street ME, Spaggiari C, Ziveri MA, Rossi M, Volta C, Viani I, et al. Insulin production and resistance in cystic fibrosis: Effect of age, disease activity, and genotype. Journal of Endocrinological Investigation. 2012;**35**(3):246-253

[36] Cano Megías M, González Albarrán O, Guisado Vasco P, Lamas Ferreiro A, Máiz CL. Insulin resistance, β-cell dysfunction and differences in curves of plasma glucose and insulin in the intermediate points of the standard glucose tolerance test in adults with cystic fibrosis. Endocrinología y Nutrición. 2015;**62**(2):91-99

[37] Tofé S, Moreno JC, Máiz L, Alonso M, Escobar H, Barrio R. Insulin-secretion abnormalities and clinical deterioration related to impaired glucose tolerance in cystic fibrosis. European Journal of Endocrinology. 2005;**152**(2):241-247

[38] Martin-Frías M, Lamas Ferreiro A, Enes Romero P, Cano Gutiérrez B, Barrio CR. Abnormal glucose tolerance in prepubertal patients with cystic fibrosis. Anales de Pediatría (Barcelona, Spain). 2012;**77**(5):339-343

[39] Mohan K, Miller H, Dyce P, Grainger R, Hughes R, Vora J, et al. Mechanisms of glucose intolerance in cystic fibrosis. Diabetic Medicine. 2009;**26**(6):582-588

[40] De Schepper J, Dab I, Derde MP, Loeb H. Oral glucose tolerance testing in cystic fibrosis: Correlations with clinical parameters and glycosylated haemoglobin determinations. European Journal of Pediatrics. 1991;**150**(6):403-406

[41] Boudreau V, Coriati A, Hammana I, Ziai S, Desjardins K, Berthiaume Y, et al. Variation of glucose tolerance in adult patients with cystic fibrosis: What is the potential contribution of insulin sensitivity? Journal of Cystic Fibrosis. 2016;**15**(6):839-845

[42] Klip A, Tsakiridis T, Marette A, Ortiz PA. Regulation of expression of glucose transporters by glucose: A review of studies in vivo and in cell cultures. The FASEB Journal. 1994;**8**(1):43-53

[43] Vuorinen-Markkola H, Koivisto VA, Yki-Jarvinen H. Mechanisms of hyperglycemia-induced insulin resistance in whole body and skeletal muscle of type I diabetic patients. Diabetes. 1992;**41**(5):571-580

[44] Hardin DS, Leblanc A, Marshall G, Seilheimer DK. Mechanisms of insulin resistance in cystic fibrosis. American Journal of Physiology. Endocrinology and Metabolism. 2001;**281**(5):E1022-E10E8

[45] Rotter V, Nagaev I, Smith U. Interleukin-6 (IL-6) induces insulin resistance in 3T3-L1 adipocytes and is, like IL-8 and tumor necrosis factor-α, overexpressed in human fat cells from insulin-resistant subjects. The Journal of Biological Chemistry. 2003;**278**(46):45777-45784

[46] Nieto-Vazquez I, Fernández-Veledo S, De Alvaro C, Lorenzo M. Dual role of interleukin-6 in regulating insulin sensitivity in murine skeletal muscle. Diabetes. 2008;**57**(12):3211-3221

[47] Hotamisligil GS, Peraldi P, Budavari A, Ellis R, White MF, Spiegelman BM. IRS-1–mediated inhibition of insulin receptor tyrosine kinase activity in TNF-α– And obesity-induced insulin resistance. Science. 1996;**271**(5249):665-668

[48] Ofei F, Hurel S, Newkirk J, Sopwith M, Taylor R. Effects of an engineered human anti–TNF-α antibody (CDP571) on insulin sensitivity and glycemic control in patients with NIDDM. Diabetes. 1996;**45**(7):881-885

[49] Amiel SA, Sherwin RS, Simonson DC, Lauritano AA, Tamborlane WV. Impaired insulin action in puberty: A contributing factor to poor glycaemic control in adolescents with diabetes. The New England Journal of Medicine. 1986;**315**(4):215-219

[50] Nezer N, Shoseyov D, Kerem E, Zangen DH. Patients with cystic fibrosis and normoglycemia exhibit diabetic glucose tolerance during pulmonary exacerbation. Journal of Cystic Fibrosis. 2010;**9**(3):199-204

[51] Iwanicki C, Logomarsino JV. Impaired glucose tolerance, body mass index and respiratory function in patients with cystic fibrosis: A systematic review. The Clinical Respiratory Journal. 2019;**13**(6):341-354

[52] Yi Y, Norris AW, Wang K, Sun X, Uc A, Moran A, et al. Abnormal glucose tolerance in infants and young children with cystic fibrosis. American Journal of Respiratory and Critical Care Medicine. 2016;**194**(8):974-980

[53] Sterescu AE, Rhodes B, Jackson R, Dupuis A, Hanna A, Wilson DC, et al. Natural history of glucose intolerance in patients with cystic fibrosis: Ten-year prospective observation program. The Journal of Pediatrics. 2010;**156**(4):613-617

[54] Lanng S, Hansen A, Thorsteinsson B, Nerup J, Koch C. Glucose tolerance in patients with cystic fibrosis: Five year prospective study. BMJ. 1995;**311**(7006):655-659

[55] Scheuing N, Holl RW, Dockter G, Hermann JM, Junge S, Koerner-Rettberg C, et al. High variability in oral glucose tolerance among 1,128 patients with cystic fibrosis: A multicenter screening study. PLoS One. 2014;**9**(11):e112578

[56] Milla CE, Billings J, Moran A. Diabetes is associated with dramatically decreased survival in female but not male subjects with cystic fibrosis. Diabetes Care. 2005;**28**(9):2141-2144

[57] Schwarzenberg SJ, Thomas W, Olsen TW, Grover T, Walk D, Milla C, et al. Microvascular complications in cystic fibrosis-related diabetes. Diabetes Care. 2007;**30**(5):1056-1061

[58] Scheuing N, Holl RW, Dockter G, Fink K, Junge S, Naehrlich L, et al. Diabetes in cystic fibrosis: Mulitcenter screening results based on current guidelines. PLoS One. 2013;**8**(12):e81545

[59] Moran A, Brunzell C, Cohen RC, Katz M, Marshall BC, Onady G, et al.

Clinical care guidelines for cystic fibrosis-related diabetes: A position statement of the American Diabetes Association and a clinical practice guideline of the Cystic Fibrosis Foundation, endorsed by the pediatric Endocrine Society. Diabetes Care. 2010;**33**(12):2697-2708

[60] Waugh N, Royle P, Craigie I, Ho V, Pandit L, Ewings P, et al. Screening for cystic fibrosis-related diabetes: A systematic review. Health Technology Assessment. 2012;**16**(24):24

[61] Hameed S, Jaffé A, Verge CF. Advances in the detection and management of cystic fibrosis related diabetes. Current Opinion in Pediatrics. 2015;**27**(4):525-533

[62] Juvenile Diabetes Research Foundation Continuous Glucose Monitoring Study Group. Continuous glucose monitoring and intensive treatment of type 1 diabetes. The New England Journal of Medicine. 2008;**359**(14):1464-1476

[63] Moran A, Becker D, Casella SJ, Gottlieb PA, Kirkman MS, Marshall BC, et al. Epidemiology, pathophysiology, and prognostic implications of cystic fibrosis-related diabetes: A technical review. Diabetes Care. 2010;**33**(12):2677-2683

[64] American Diabetes Association. Classification and diagnosis of diabetes: Standards of medical care in diabetes. Diabetes Care. 2020;**43**:S14-S31

[65] Juvenile Diabetes Research Foundation Continuous Glucose Monitoring Study Group. Variation of interstitial glucose measurements assessed by continuous glucose monitors in healthy, nondiabetic individuals. Diabetes Care. 2010;**33**(6):1297-1299

[66] Noronha RM, Damaceno N, Muramatu LH, Monte O, Calliari LEP. Importance of screening with oral glucose tolerance test for early diagnosis of cystic fibrosis-related diabetes mellitus. Pediatric Diabetes. 2014;**15**(4):309-312

[67] Middleton PG, Wagenaar M, Matson AG, Craig ME, Holmes-Walker DJ, Katz T, et al. Australian standards of care for cystic fibrosis-related diabetes. Respirology. 2014;**19**(2):185-192

[68] Yung B, Kemp M, Hooper J, Hodson ME. Diagnosis of cystic fibrosis related diabetes: A selective approach in performing the oral glucose tolerance test based on a combination of clinical and biochemical criteria. Thorax. 1999;**54**(1):40-43

[69] Widger J, Hameed S, Ooi CY, Verge C. Using HbA1c as a screening tool for cystic fibrosis related diabetes. Journal of Cystic Fibrosis. 2016;**15**(2):263-264

[70] Garagorri JM, Rodriguez G, Ros L, Sanchez A. Early detection of impaired glucose tolerance in patients with cystic fibrosis and predisposition factors. Journal of Pediatric Endocrinology & Metabolism. 2001;**14**(1):53-60

[71] Coriati A, Ziai S, Azar M, Berthiaume Y, Rabasa-Lhoret R. Characterization of patients with cystic fibrosis presenting an indeterminate glucose tolerance (INDET). Journal of Cystic Fibrosis. 2016;**15**(1):127-132

[72] Lavie M, Fisher D, Vilozni D, Forschmidt R, Sarouk I, Kanety H, et al. Glucose intolerance in cystic fibrosis as a determinant of pulmonary function and clinical status. Diabetes Research and Clinical Practice. 2015;**110**(3):276-284

[73] Franzese A, Valerio G, Buono P, Spagnuolo MI, Sepe A, Mozzillo E, et al. Continuous glucose monitoring system in the screening of early glucose derangements in children and adolescents with cystic fibrosis.

Journal of Pediatric Endocrinology & Metabolism. 2008;**21**(2):109-116

[74] Tommerdahl KL, Brinton JT, Vigers T, Nadeau KJ, Zeitler PS, Chan CL. Screening for cystic fibrosis-related diabetes and prediabetes: Evaluating 1,5-anhydroglucitol, fructosamine, glycated albumin, and hemoglobin A1c. Pediatric Diabetes. 2019;**20**(8):1080-1086

[75] Chan CL, Hope E, Thurston J, Vigers T, Pyle L, Zeitler PS, et al. Hemoglobin A1c accurately predicts continuous glucose monitoring–derived average glucose in youth and young adults with cystic fibrosis. Diabetes Care. 2018;**41**(7):1406-1413

[76] Godbout A, Hammana I, Potvin S, Mainville D, Rakel A, Berthiaume Y, et al. No relationship between mean plasma glucose and glycated haemoglobin in patients with cystic fibrosis-related diabetes. Diabetes & Metabolism. 2008;**34**(6):568-573

[77] Rana M, Munns CF, Selvadurai H, Donaghue KC, Craig ME. Cystic fibrosis-related diabetes in children—Gaps in the evidence? Nature Reviews. Endocrinology. 2010;**6**(7):371-378

[78] Prentice B, Hameed S, Verge CF, Ooi CY, Jaffe A, Widger J. Diagnosing cystic fibrosis-related diabetes: Current methods and challenges. Expert Review of Respiratory Medicine. 2016;**10**(7):799-811

[79] Brennan AL, Gyi KM, Wood DM, Hodson ME, Geddes DM, Baker EH. Relationship between glycosylated haemoglobin and mean plasma glucose concentration in cystic fibrosis. Journal of Cystic Fibrosis. 2006;**5**(1):27-31

[80] De Luca F, Arrigo T, Nibali SC, Sferlazzas C, Gigante A, Di Cesare E, et al. Insulin secretion, glycosylated haemoglobin and islet cell antibodies in cystic fibrosis children and adolescents with different degrees of glucose tolerance. Hormone and Metabolic Research. 1991;**23**(10):495-498

[81] Rana M, Munns CF, Selvadurai HC, Simonds S, Cooper PJ, Woodhead HJ, et al. Increased detection of cystic-fibrosis-related diabetes in Australia. Archives of Disease in Childhood. 2011;**96**(9):823-826

[82] Burgess JC, Bridges N, Banya W, Gyi KM, Hodson ME, Bilton D, et al. HbA1c as a screening tool for cystic fibrosis related diabetes. Journal of Cystic Fibrosis. 2016;**15**(2):251-257

[83] Coriati A, Elisha B, Virassamynaik S, Phaneuf M, Ziai S, Gauthier M-S, et al. Diagnosis of cystic fibrosis-related glucose abnormalities: Can we shorten the standard oral glucose tolerance test? Applied Physiology, Nutrition, and Metabolism. 2013;**38**(12):1254-1259

[84] Boudreau V, Lehoux Dubois C, Desjardins K, Mailhot M, Tremblay F, Rabasa-Lhoret R. Sensitivity and specificity of cystic fibrosis-related diabetes screening methods: Which test should be the reference method? Journal of Pediatric Endocrinology & Metabolism. 2017;**30**(8):885-887

[85] Clemente León M, Bilbao Gassó L, Moreno-Galdó A, Campos Martorrell A, Gartner Tizzano S, Yeste Fernández D, et al. Oral glucose tolerance test and continuous glucose monitoring to assess diabetes development in cystic fibrosis patients. Endocrinología, Diabetes y Nutrición. 2018;**65**(1):45-51

[86] Lam GY, Sissons S, Smith MP, Brown NE, Leung WM, Estey MP. How reliable is your HbA1c test? Revisiting the use of HbA1c in cystic fibrosis-related diabetes (CFRD) screening. Journal of Cystic Fibrosis. 2019;**18**(2):e14-e15

[87] Peckham D. Routine screening for cystic fibrosis-related diabetes. Journal

of the Royal Society of Medicine. 2009;**102**:36-39

[88] Solomon MP, Wilson DC, Corey M, Kalnins D, Zielenski J, Tsui LC, et al. Glucose intolerance in children with cystic fibrosis. The Journal of Pediatrics. 2003;**142**(2):128-132

[89] Lee KMN, Miller RJH, Rosenberg FM, Kreisman SH. Evaluation of glucose tolerance in cystic fibrosis: Comparison of 50-g and 75-g tests. Journal of Cystic Fibrosis. 2007;**6**(4):274-276

[90] Choudhury M, Taylor P, Morgan PH, Duckers J, Lau D, George L, et al. Association between HbA 1c and the development of cystic fibrosis-related diabetes. Diabetic Medicine. 2019;**36**(10):1251-1255

[91] Moran A, Hardin D, Rodman D, Allen HF, Beall RJ, Borowitz D, et al. Diagnosis, screening and management of cystic fibrosis related diabetes mellitus. Diabetes Research and Clinical Practice. 1999;**45**(1):61-73

[92] Moran A, Pekow P, Grover P, Zorn M, Slovis B, Pilewski J, et al. Insulin therapy to improve BMI in cystic fibrosis-related diabetes without fasting hyperglycemia: Results of the cystic fibrosis related diabetes therapy trial. Diabetes Care. 2009;**32**(10):1783-1788

[93] Ode KL, Frohnert B, Laguna T, Phillips J, Holme B, Regelmann W, et al. Oral glucose tolerance testing in children with cystic fibrosis. Pediatric Diabetes. 2010;**11**(7):487-492

[94] Mueller-Brandes C. New criteria for impaired fasting glucose and screening for diabetes in cystic fibrosis. The European Respiratory Journal. 2005;**25**(4):715-717

[95] Frohnert BI, Ode KL, Moran A, Nathan BM, Laguna T, Holme B, et al. Impaired fasting glucose in cystic fibrosis. Diabetes Care. 2010;**33**(12):2660-2664

[96] Schmid K, Fink K, Holl RW, Hebestreit H, Ballmann M. Predictors for future cystic fibrosis-related diabetes by oral glucose tolerance test. Journal of Cystic Fibrosis. 2014;**13**(1):80-85

[97] Boudreau V, Reynaud Q, Dubois CL, Coriati A, Desjardins K, Durieu I, et al. Screening for cystic fibrosis-related diabetes: Matching pathophysiology and addressing current challenges. Canadian Journal of Diabetes. 2016;**40**(5):466-470

[98] Taylor-Cousar JL, Janssen JS, Wilson A, Clair CG, Pickard KM, Jones MC, et al. Glucose >200 mg/dL during continuous glucose monitoring identifies adult patients at risk for development of cystic fibrosis related diabetes. Journal Diabetes Research. 2016;**2016**:1527932

[99] Gilmour JA, Sykes J, Etchells E, Tullis E. Cystic fibrosis-related diabetes screening in adults: A gap analysis and evaluation of accuracy of glycated hemoglobin levels. Canadian Journal of Diabetes. 2019;**43**(1):13-18

[100] Cystic Fibrosis Foundation Patient Registry. Annual data report. Bethesda MD: Cystic Fibrosis Foundation; 2018

[101] Sheikh S, Localio AR, Kelly A, Rubenstein RC. Abnormal glucose tolerance and the 50-gram glucose challenge test in cystic fibrosis. Journal of Cystic Fibrosis. 2020. (Forthcoming). DOI: 10.1016/j.jcf.2020.01.003

[102] Chase HP, Beck R, Tamborlane W, Buckingham B, Mauras N, Tsalikian E, et al. A randomized multicenter trial comparing the GlucoWatch biographer with standard glucose monitoring in children with type 1 diabetes. Diabetes Care. 2005;**28**(5):1101-1106

[103] Chan CL, Ode KL, Granados A, Moheet A, Moran A, Hameed S.

Continuous glucose monitoring in cystic fibrosis – A practical guide. Journal of Cystic Fibrosis. 2019;**18**:S25-S31

[104] O'Riordan SM, Hindmarsh P, Hill NR, Matthews DR, George S, Greally P, et al. Validation of continuous glucose monitoring in children and adolescents with cystic fibrosis: A prospective cohort study. Diabetes Care. 2009;**32**(6):1020-1022

[105] Dobson L, Sheldon CD, Hattersley AT. Validation of interstitial fluid continuous glucose monitoring in cystic fibrosis. Diabetes Care. 2003;**26**(6):1940-1941

[106] Dobson L, Sheldon CD, Hattersley AT. Conventional measures underestimate glycaemia in cystic fibrosis patients. Diabetic Medicine. 2004;**21**(7):691-696

[107] Schiaffini R, Brufani C, Russo B, Fintini D, Migliaccio A, Pecorelli L, et al. Abnormal glucose tolerance in children with cystic fibrosis: The predictive role of continuous glucose monitoring system. European Journal of Endocrinology. 2010;**162**(4):705-710

[108] Pu MZMH, Gonçalves AC, Minnicucci WJ, Morcillo AM, Ribeiro JD, Ribeiro AF. Continuous glucose monitoring to evaluate glycaemic abnormalities in cystic fibrosis. Archives of Disease in Childhood. 2018;**103**(6):592-596

[109] Soliman A, DeSanctis V, Yassin M, Elalaily R, Eldarsy N. Continuous glucose monitoring system and new era of early diagnosis of diabetes in high risk groups. Indian Journal of Endocrinology and Metabolism. 2014;**18**(3):274-282

[110] Ahmed MI, Fox R, Shinkins B, Sutton S, Tziaferi V, Gaillard EA. Continuous glucose monitoring systems for the diagnosis of cystic fibrosis-related diabetes (protocol). Cochrane Database of Systematic Reviews. 2018;**2018**(2):CD012953

[111] Brugha R, Wright M, Nolan S, Bridges N, Carr SB. Quantifying fluctuation in glucose levels to identify early changes in glucose homeostasis in cystic fibrosis. Journal of Cystic Fibrosis. 2018;**17**(6):791-797

[112] Frost F, Dyce P, Nazareth D, Malone V, Walshaw MJ. Continuous glucose monitoring guided insulin therapy is associated with improved clinical outcomes in cystic fibrosis-related diabetes. Journal of Cystic Fibrosis. 2018;**17**(6):798-803

[113] Granados A, Chan CL, Ode KL, Moheet A, Moran A, Holl R. Cystic fibrosis related diabetes: Pathophysiology, screening and diagnosis. Journal of Cystic Fibrosis. 2019;**18**:S3-S9

[114] Andersen HU, Lanng S, Pressler T, Laugesen CS, Mathiesen ER. Cystic fibrosis-related diabetes: The presence of microvascular diabetes complications. Diabetes Care. 2006;**29**(12):2660-2663

[115] Van Den Berg JMW, Morton AM, Kok SW, Pijl H, Conway SP, Heijerman HGM. Microvascular complications in patients with cystic fibrosis-related diabetes (CFRD). Journal of Cystic Fibrosis. 2008;**7**(6):515-519

[116] Okoniewski W, Hughan KS, Weiner GA, Weiner DJ, Forno E. Glycemic control and FEV1 recovery during pulmonary exacerbations in pediatric cystic fibrosis-related diabetes. Journal of Cystic Fibrosis. 2020. (Forthcoming). DOI: 10.1016/j.jcf.2019.12.016

[117] Olesen HV, Drevinek P, Gulmans VA, Hatziagorou E, Jung A, Mei-Zahav M, et al. Cystic fibrosis related diabetes in Europe: Prevalence,

risk factors and outcome. Journal of Cystic Fibrosis. 2020;**19**(2):321-327

[118] Miller RJ, Tildesley HD, Wilcox PG, Zhang H, Kreisman SH. Sex disparities in effects of cystic fibrosis-related diabetes on clinical outcomes: A matched study. Canadian Respiratory Journal. 2008;**15**(6):291-294

[119] Sharma R, Florea VG, Bolger AP, Doehner W, Florea ND, Coats AJ, et al. Wasting as an independent predictor of mortality in patients with cystic fibrosis. Thorax. 2001;**56**(10):746-750

[120] Belle-van Meerkerk G, de Valk HW, Stam-Slob MC, Teding van Berkhout F, Zanen P, van de Graaf EA. Cystic fibrosis-related diabetes with strict glycaemic control is not associated with frequent intravenous antibiotics use for pulmonary infections. Diabetes Research and Clinical Practice. 2016;**116**:230-236

[121] Van Sambeek L, Cowley ES, Newman DK, Kato R. Sputum glucose and glycemic control in cystic fibrosis-related diabetes: A cross-sectional study. PLoS One. 2015;**10**(3):e0119938

[122] Mozzillo E, Franzese A, Valerio G, Sepe A, De Simone I, Mazzarella G, et al. One-year glargine treatment can improve the course of lung disease in children and adolescents with cystic fibrosis and early glucose derangements. Pediatric Diabetes. 2009;**10**(3):162-167

[123] Wooldridge JL, Szczesniak RD, Fenchel MC, Elder DA. Insulin secretion abnormalities in exocrine pancreatic sufficient cystic fibrosis patients. Journal of Cystic Fibrosis. 2015;**14**(6):792-797

[124] Alicandro G, Battezzati PM, Battezzati A, Speziali C, Claut L, Motta V, et al. Insulin secretion, nutritional status and respiratory function in cystic fibrosis patients with normal glucose tolerance. Clinical Nutrition. 2012;**31**(1):118-123

[125] Brennan AL, Gyi KM, Wood DM, Johnson J, Holliman R, Baines DL, et al. Airway glucose concentrations and effect on growth of respiratory pathogens in cystic fibrosis. Journal of Cystic Fibrosis. 2007;**6**(2):101-109

[126] Gill SK, Hui K, Farne H, Garnett JP, Baines DL, Moore LSP, et al. Increased airway glucose increases airway bacterial load in hyperglycaemia. Scientific Reports. 2016;**6**(1):27636

[127] Garnett JP, Kalsi KK, Sobotta M, Bearham J, Carr G, Powell J, et al. Hyperglycaemia and Pseudomonas aeruginosa acidify cystic fibrosis airway surface liquid by elevating epithelial monocarboxylate transporter 2 dependent lactate-H+ secretion. Scientific Reports. 2016;**6**:37955

[128] Baker EH, Clark N, Brennan AL, Fisher DA, Gyi KM, Hodson ME, et al. Hyperglycemia and cystic fibrosis alter respiratory fluid glucose concentrations estimated by breath condensate analysis. Journal of Applied Physiology. 2007;**102**(5):1969-1975

[129] Garnett JP, Gray MA, Tarran R, Brodlie M, Ward C, Baker EH, et al. Elevated paracellular glucose flux across cystic fibrosis airway epithelial monolayers is an important factor for Pseudomonas aeruginosa growth. PLoS One. 2013;**8**(10):e76283

[130] Philips BJ, Redman J, Brennan A, Wood D, Holliman R, Baines D, et al. Glucose in bronchial aspirates increases the risk of respiratory MRSA in intubated patients. Thorax. 2005;**60**(9):761-764

[131] Merlo CA, Boyle MP, Diener-West M, Marshall BC, Goss CH, Lechtzin N. Incidence and risk factors for multiple antibiotic-resistant Pseudomonas aeruginosa in cystic fibrosis. Chest. 2007;**132**(2):562-568

[132] Frost F, Nazareth D, Shaw M, Walshaw MJ. Cystic fibrosis related

diabetes is not independently associated with increased Stenotrophomonas maltophilia infection: Longitudinal data from the UK CF registry. Journal of Cystic Fibrosis. 2019;**18**(2):294-298

[133] Ziegler B, Oliveira CL, Rovedder PM, Schuh SJ. Abreu e Silva FA, de Tarso Roth Dalcin P. glucose intolerance in patients with cystic fibrosis: Sex-based differences in clinical score, pulmonary function, radiograph score, and 6-minute walk test. Respiratory Care. 2011;**56**(3):290-297

[134] van den Borst B, Gosker HR, Zeegers MP, Schols AM. Pulmonary function in diabetes: A metaanalysis. Chest. 2010;**138**(2):393-406

[135] Konstan MW, Hilliard KA, Norvell TM, Berger M. Bronchoalveolar lavage findings in cystic fibrosis patients with stable, clinically mild lung disease suggest ongoing infection and inflammation. American Journal of Respiratory and Critical Care Medicine. 1994;**150**(2):448-454

[136] Bruce MC, Poncz L, Klinger JD, Stern RC, Tomashefski JF Jr, Dearborn DG. Biochemical and pathologic evidence for proteolytic destruction of lung connective tissue in cystic fibrosis. The American Review of Respiratory Disease. 1985;**132**(3):529-535

[137] Ntimbane T, Krishnamoorthy P, Huot C, Legault L, Jacob SV, Brunet S, et al. Oxidative stress and cystic fibrosis-related diabetes: A pilot study in children. Journal of Cystic Fibrosis. 2008;**7**(5):373-384

[138] Arora NS, Rochester DF. Respiratory muscle strength and maximal voluntary ventilation in undernourished patients. The American Review of Respiratory Disease. 1982;**126**(1):5-8

[139] Arora NS, Rochester DF. Effect of body weight and muscularity on human diaphragm muscle mass, thickness, and area. Journal of Applied Physiology. 1982;**52**(1):64-70

[140] Konstan MW, Morgan WJ, Butler SM, Pasta DJ, Craib ML, Silva SJ, et al. Risk factors for rate of decline in forced expiratory volume in one second in children and adolescents with cystic fibrosis. The Journal of Pediatrics. 2007;**151**(2):134-139

[141] Sanders DB, Emerson J, Ren CL, Schechter MS, Gibson RL, Morgan W, et al. Early childhood risk factors for decreased FEV1 at age six to seven years in young children with cystic fibrosis. Annals of the American Thoracic Society. 2015;**12**(8):1170-1176

[142] Coderre L, Fadainia C, Belson L, Belisle V, Ziai S, Maillhot G, et al. LDL-cholesterol and insulin are independently associated with body mass index in adult cystic fibrosis patients. Journal of Cystic Fibrosis. 2012;**11**(5):393-397

[143] Bizzarri C, Lucidi V, Ciampalini P, Bella S, Russo B, Cappa M. Clinical effects of early treatment with insulin glargine in patients with cystic fibrosis and impaired glucose tolerance. Journal of Endocrinological Investigation. 2006;**29**(3):RC1-RC4

[144] Bizzarri C, Montemitro E, Pedicelli S, Ciccone S, Majo F, Cappa M, et al. Glucose tolerance affects pubertal growth and final height of children with cystic fibrosis. Pediatric Pulmonology. 2015;**50**(2):144-149

[145] Cheung MS, Bridges NA, Prasad SA, Francis J, Carr SB, Suri R, et al. Growth in children with cystic fibrosis-related diabetes. Pediatric Pulmonology. 2009;**44**(12):1223-1225

[146] Terliesner N, Vogel M, Steighardt A, Gausche R, Henn C, Hentschel J, et al. Cystic-fibrosis related-diabetes (CFRD) is preceded by

and associated with growth failure and deteriorating lung function. Journal of Pediatric Endocrinology & Metabolism. 2017;**30**(8):815-821

[147] White H, Pollard K, Etherington C, Clifton I, Morton AM, Owen D, et al. Nutritional decline in cystic fibrosis related diabetes: The effect of intensive nutritional intervention. Journal of Cystic Fibrosis. 2009;**8**(3):179-185

[148] Bennett P, Burch T, Miller M. Diabetes mellitus in American (Pima) Indians. The Lancet. 1971;**298**(7716):125-128

[149] Olszowiec-Chlebna M, Koniarek-Maniecka A, Stelmach W, Smejda K, Jerzyńska J, Majak P, et al. Predictors of deterioration of lung function in polish children with cystic fibrosis. Archives of Medical Science. 2016;**2**:402-407

[150] Coriati A, Ziai S, Lavoie A, Berthiaume Y, Rabasa-Lhoret R. The 1-h oral glucose tolerance test glucose and insulin values are associated with markers of clinical deterioration in cystic fibrosis. Acta Diabetologica. 2016;**53**(3):359-366

[151] Bourdy S, Rabilloud M, Touzet S, Roche S, Drai J, Martin C, et al. 178 glucose tolerance in cystic fibrosis patients over a 3-year period (DIAMUCO study). Journal of Cystic Fibrosis. 2015;**14**:S103

[152] Chan CL, Vigers T, Pyle L, Zeitler PS, Sagel SD, Nadeau KJ. Continuous glucose monitoring abnormalities in cystic fibrosis youth correlate with pulmonary function decline. Journal of Cystic Fibrosis. 2018;**17**(6):783-790

[153] Prentice BJ, Chelliah A, Ooi CY, Hameed S, Verge CF, Plush L, et al. Peak OGTT glucose is associated with lower lung function in young children with cystic fibrosis. Journal of Cystic Fibrosis. 2020;**19**(2):305-309

[154] Reynaud Q, Rabilloud M, Roche S, Poupon-Bourdy S, Iwaz J, Nove-Josserand R, et al. Glucose trajectories in cystic fibrosis and their association with pulmonary function. Journal of Cystic Fibrosis. 2018;**17**(3):400-406

[155] Leclercq A, Gauthier B, Rosner V, Weiss L, Moreau F, Constantinescu AA, et al. Early assessment of glucose abnormalities during continuous glucose monitoring associated with lung function impairment in cystic fibrosis patients. Journal of Cystic Fibrosis. 2014;**13**(4):478-484

[156] Prentice BJ, Ooi CY, Strachan RE, Hameed S, Ebrahimkhani S, Waters SA, et al. Early glucose abnormalities are associated with pulmonary inflammation in young children with cystic fibrosis. Journal of Cystic Fibrosis. 2019;**18**(6):869-873

[157] Lam GY, Doll-Shankaruk M, Dayton J, Rodriguez-Capote K, Higgins TN, Thomas D, et al. The use of fructosamine in cystic fibrosis-related diabetes (CFRD) screening. Journal of Cystic Fibrosis. 2018;**17**(1):121-124

[158] Onady GM, Stolfi A. Insulin and oral agents for managing cystic fibrosis-related diabetes. Cochrane Database of Systematic Reviews. 2016;**4**:CD004730

[159] Barrio R. Cystic fibrosis-related diabetes: Novel pathogenic insights opening new therapeutic avenues. European Journal of Endocrinology. 2015;**172**(4):R131-RR41

[160] Bellin MD, Laguna T, Leschyshyn J, Regelmann W, Dunitz J, Billings J, et al. Insulin secretion improves in cystic fibrosis following ivacaftor correction of CFTR: A small pilot study. Pediatric Diabetes. 2013;**14**(6):417-421

[161] Kelly A, De Leon DD, Sheikh S, Camburn D, Kubrak C, Peleckis AJ, et al. Islet hormone and incretin secretion in cystic fibrosis after four

months of ivacaftor therapy. American Journal of Respiratory and Critical Care Medicine. 2019;**199**(3):342-351

[162] Minicucci L, Haupt M, Casciaro R, De Alessandri A, Bagnasco F, Lucidi V, et al. Slow-release insulin in cystic fibrosis patients with glucose intolerance: A randomized clinical trial. Pediatric Diabetes. 2012;**13**(2):197-202

[163] Kolouskova S, Zemkova D, Bartosova J, Skalicka V, Sumnik Z, Vavrova V, et al. Low-dose insulin therapy in patients with cystic fibrosis and early-stage insulinopenia prevents deterioration of lung function: A 3-year prospective study. Journal of Pediatric Endocrinology & Metabolism. 2011;**24**(7-8):449-454

[164] Drummond RS, Ross E, Bicknell S, Small M, Jones GC. Insulin therapy in patients with cystic fibrosis related diabetes mellitus: Benefit, timing of initiation and hypoglycaemia. Practical Diabetes International. 2011;**28**(4):177-182

[165] Hameed S, Morton JR, Field PI, Belessis Y, Yoong T, Katz T, et al. Once daily insulin detemir in cystic fibrosis with insulin deficiency. Archives of Disease in Childhood. 2012;**97**(5):464-467

[166] Pu MZMH, Christensen-Adad FC, Gonçalves AC, Minicucci WJ, Ribeiro JD, Ribeiro AF. Insulin therapy in patients with cystic fibrosis in the pre-diabetes stage: A systematic review. Revista Paulista de Pediatria. 2016;**34**(3):367-373

Chapter 4

Microbial Cystic Fibrosis

Waleed Mohamed Abdulkhair and
Mousa Abdullah Alghuthaymi

Abstract

Cystic fibrosis (CF) is the most common genetic disease in Caucasians that increases the mortality rate. This disease retards the passage of water and salt through the cells and therefore affects the vital functions of different organs. Pulmonary cystic fibrosis is the most common and responsible for the majority of symptoms, burden of care, and mortality. The gene that causes the disease has now been identified and sequenced. The lung diseases with CF are usually have three pathological elements; mucus obstruction, inflammation, and infection. In the last century, the relationship between CF, respiratory microbiology, and inflammation has been understood with increased longevity and development of new treatments and laboratory techniques. In this chapter, we will illustrate causes of CF lung diseases and modern therapeutic strategies.

Keywords: cystic fibrosis, pathogenic bacteria, pneumonia infection, pulmonary inflammation, treatment guidelines

1. Introduction

Cystic fibrosis (CF) arises due to recessive mutations in the CF transmembrane regulator (CFTR) gene. This genetic disorder is carried out when two carrier parents transport the mutant CFTR gene to their child. Although no symptoms appear in the carriers, CF can be detected by genetic testing. CF-pulmonary diseases are usually associated with three pathological aspects; airway obstruction, infection, and inflammation. According to previous studies, children are most frequently infected by this disease with high rate of mortality. *Staphylococcus aureus* is the main cause of bronchitis, bronchiectasis, and pulmonary abscesses arising in the bronchi, which are usually accompanied by tenacious greenish-gray mucopurulent material [1, 2].

The mutation that attacks CFTR gene leads to CF, and obstruction in the airways with abnormal mucus, infection, and inflammation is present. Although the current treatments cannot halt the disease progression, good nutrition, defective mucus clearance, and treatment of inflammation and infection greatly improve CF of the respiratory system and its complications [3]. There is a controversial relationship between infection and inflammation. Some scientists think that the infection should precede the inflammation of airways, while others suggest the opposite [4].

Americans and Europeans are more susceptible to CF. One in 29 people of Caucasian ancestry is a healthy carrier of the CF gene mutation [5]. Detection of CF in early phases is very useful due to symptom reduction, health improvement, and low cost. For example, since 2010s, all American newborns undergo screening for CF to provide a chance for recovery if the disease is diagnosed. Most patients of CF must take pancreatic enzymes to digest food effectively, and some require insulin for diabetes mellitus. The treatment cost of CF is very high because the drugs which treat and prevent the pulmonary diseases are very expensive [6]. Walaa et al. [7] report that 60 Egyptian children are affected by CF (6 months to 14 years). Salty skin is the most common symptom in the children affected with CF, because they suffer from dehydration due to loss of exuberant salty sweat. The percentage of ill males is 63%, while the percentage of ill females is 37%. Positive consanguinity of patients is 57%. 23% of patients has a positive family history of CF; the most frequent clinical presentation is pulmonary disease (84%), followed by pancreatic insufficiency (56%). The scientific material of this chapter aims to clearly interpret the roles of infection and inflammation in CF lung disease pathogenesis. Also, we will shed light on the therapeutic approaches to both infection and inflammation.

2. Microbes: CF interaction

2.1 Microbiology of CF lung disease

Severe and uncontrolled microbial infection may lead to CF. Microbes usually invade the airway luminal mucus, rather than tissues. Although *Staphylococcus aureus* is the main pathogenic agent for CF, many other bacteria are recorded with the development of both treatments and laboratory methods. The detection of pathogenic bacteria of CF depends on the cultivation of respiratory samples (e.g., sputum, bronchoalveolar lavage fluid, oropharyngeal swabs, or sinus samples) on the nutritive and selective media. Moreover, there are advanced techniques by which CF microbes are identified. Current methods mainly depend on cultivation of pathogenic bacteria on synthetic microbiological growth media and follow the incubation conditions to allow good growth and culture characteristics of pathogens [8]. Conventional techniques including microscopic and biochemical investigations revealed that the pathogenic microbes infecting CF airways usually exist in biofilms, which provide complete defense mechanism to the pathogens [9, 10].

2.2 CF respiratory pathogens

2.2.1 Staphylococcus aureus

Staphylococcus aureus is a Gram-positive bacterium and is the first CF respiratory pathogen. Children are more susceptible to CF lung diseases than adults, and they are usually affected by *S. aureus*, which has been associated with higher airway inflammation [11, 12] and lung dysfunctions [13, 14]. This infection can be lethal when associated with *Pseudomonas aeruginosa* [15]. This association may lead to worse outcomes, if *P. aeruginosa* is associated with specific subtypes of *S. aureus* such as methicillin-resistant *S. aureus* (MRSA) and small-colony variants of *S. aureus* (SCVs). *S. aureus* infection in adults is harmless than in children, because lung functions are better [16] and there are lower complications [17]. Accordingly, the pathogenicity of *S. aureus* has two levels: the first is high when the infection occurs in children or in the absence of *P. aeruginosa*, and the second is very high (extreme) when the host is infected by specific subtypes of *S. aureus* (such as MRSA or SCVs). On the other hand, *S. aureus* may be nonpathogenic, but just serves as a marker of early or mild disease as with children and adults, respectively [18].

The two subtypes of *S. aureus* which are mentioned above (MRSA and SCVs) as well as oxacillin-resistant *S. aureus* (ORSA) are usually identified either by their resistance to these β-lactams or by carriage of the *mec*A gene, which encodes this resistance. The subtypes of *S. aureus* SCVs are slow-growing, antibiotic-resistant variants that are difficult to detect with conventional cultures and require special laboratory methods. SCVs are associated with decreasing lung functions, and they may be treated with antibiotics including aminoglycosides and sulfonamides [19]. MRSA are tightly accompanied with CF lung disease especially in the last 20 years. A lot of people are infected with MRSA due to hospitalization and worse use of antibiotics [20–22]. Many studies reported that MRSA are associated with CF lung disease in particular decrease of lung functions [23]. Moreover, MRSA is an independent risk factor for decreasing lung functions and respiratory exacerbations [24] and for increased mortality [25]. There are some similarities between the two subtypes (MRSA and SCVs): antibiotic treatment, antibiotic resistance, and higher lung disease severity.

In some countries where CF lung disease is spreading, anti-staphylococcal agent is provided as a prophylaxis approach during childhood particularly when *P. aeruginosa* is detected early [26]. Many of antibiotics are used to eradicate *S. aureus* and *P. aeruginosa* as co-infectious agents of CF lung disease, but the most commonly used antibiotics are aminoglycosides and sulfonamides [27].

2.2.2 *Pseudomonas aeruginosa*

After overcoming *S. aureus* by effective anti-staphylococcal agents, *P. aeruginosa* became the most common and important pathogen related to CF-pulmonary diseases [28]. *P. aeruginosa* infection is associated with decreasing lung functions, severe inflammation of the respiratory tract, a greater risk of respiratory exacerbations, and high rate of mortality [29]. Early detection of *P. aeruginosa* is a helpful factor for full eradication, while chronic infection cannot be eradicated. Also, eradication of *P. aeruginosa* can be carried out by using antipseudomonal bioagents [30]. In contrast with *S. aureus* infection, *P. aeruginosa* infection is higher in adults than in children. At the end-stage of CF-pulmonary disease, *P. aeruginosa* is only present as a main pathogen for respiratory tract 31].

Despite *P. aeruginosa* usually producing numerous toxins as virulence factors, it may loss these virulence factors or their regulatory genes during chronic CF infections [32]. After invasion of lungs with *P. aeruginosa*, the mucoid colonies are formed due to exuberant production of alginate as one of the phenotypic changes due to chronic infection of CF-pulmonary disease [33]. The mucoid texture provides high rates of persistence and resistance for many antimicrobial agents as well as full adaptation to the respiratory airways. *P. aeruginosa* may be epidemic or non-epidemic, but the former is associated with worse outcomes such as high rate of mortality and requirement for lung transplantation [34].

Although *P. aeruginosa* is a multidrug resistant pathogen and usually leads to severe pulmonary CF, it leads to worse outcomes when associated with MRSA and SCVs. Prophylaxis by using of antibiotics is not recommended in the recent approach of *P. aeruginosa* treatment due to severe adverse events of antibiotics, but if *P. aeruginosa* is early detected, the treatment course with antibiotics must begin for complete eradication and to decrease the risk of exacerbations. Recently, inhaled antibiotics such as tobramycin and aztreonam are sufficient for eradication without any additional oral antibiotics such as ciprofloxacin [35]. Although inhaled antibiotics are sufficient for *P. aeruginosa* treatment without oral antibiotics, the clinical reports are revealing that, the combination between two classes of antibiotics leads to longer periods of clinical stability than does a single class [36].

2.2.3 *Burkholderia cepacia complex*

Burkholderia cepacia complex (BCC) is a group of Gram-negative bacteria and is comprised of at least 18 species. Of these, two species are the most common and associated with CF lung infections and disease, *B. cenocepacia* and *B. multivorans*, but the latter is more distributed than the former. Nevertheless, *B. cenocepacia* is associated with more rapid lung function decline and mortality rate than *B. multivorans*. Other BCC species are less common, and their clinical associations are less well defined such as *B. gladioli* [37]. *Burkholderia* CF infections are notorious because they are associated with more severe lung disease, they are transmissible among persons with CF, they are resistant to multi-antibiotics, and epidemic strains can infect CF patients after internal contact at camps and clinics [38]. Associated outcomes often range from clinical quiescence to rapidly progressive, necrotizing pneumonia and fatal septic disease "cepacia syndrome" [39]. Therapy is usually limited to specific antibiotics as needed [40, 41].

2.2.4 *Stenotrophomonas maltophilia*

Stenotrophomonas maltophilia is a Gram-negative bacterium, which is widely spreading in the United States in recent years as CF pathogen especially among adolescents and young adults. This bacterium has intrinsic and acquired resistance to many antibiotics. No clear evidence for treatment of this pathogen so far [42].

2.2.5 *Haemophilus influenzae*

Haemophilus influenzae is a Gram-negative bacterium and is firstly detected in CF respiratory cultures. This bacterium is more prevalent in children and less common in adults. Although its association with CF complications is controversial, it is associated with non-CF bronchiectasis and chronic obstructive pulmonary disease. The cultivation of this bacterium is difficult and usually requires specific conditions for detection. The recent isolates of *H. influenzae* are non-typeable and unencapsulated since the vaccine of *H. influenzae* type B (HIB) has been discovered. This bacterium is well known as resistant to β-lactam antibiotics due to its production of β-lactamase; therefore, treatments usually include a β-lactamase inhibitor such as amoxicillin-clavulanate [43].

2.2.6 *Achromobacter xylosoxidans*

Achromobacter xylosoxidans is a Gram-negative bacterium that is similar to *P. aeruginosa*. Although this bacterium is widely spreading in the United States, it remains low in CF lung diseases (<10%). This bacterium is associated with worse radiographic and spirometric measures of lung disease. Similar to *P. aeruginosa* and BCC, *A. xylosoxidans* is the dominant, and occasionally, bacterium is isolated from CF patients at end-stage. Some microbes are notorious due to their resistance to many antibiotics, so their treatment is limited [44].

2.2.7 *Nontuberculous mycobacteria*

Nontuberculous mycobacteria represent 6–30% of CF prevalence. Two groups of mycobacteria, accounting for six species, are currently considered important CF pathogens: *Mycobacterium avium* and *Mycobacterium abscessus* complexes. The treatment of nontuberculous mycobacteria has two phases: multiple intravenous antibiotics for weeks to months or multiple inhaled and oral antibiotics for months to years. Side-effects and toxicities are common and can be troublesome [45].

2.2.8 *Fungi and viruses*

A lot of fungi are isolated from CF patients, including yeasts such as *Candida* spp. and filamentous fungi such as *Aspergillus* spp. There is a respiratory disease known as allergic bronchopulmonary aspergillosis (ABPA), in which the bronchia are affected by inflammation due to *Aspergillus* infection. Patients of CF and other chronic airway diseases can develop an IgE-mediated allergic airway disease known as ABPA. The treatment for which primarily involves steroids, although the addition of an antifungal such as itraconazole may allow for lower doses of steroids. Human respiratory viruses are not thought to chronically infect the CF airway, but they have been shown both to be important and common triggers of CF respiratory exacerbations [45].

2.3 CF airway microbiome

Many studies which are concerned with identification of the microbiota of the respiratory system depend on DNA-sequencing techniques. The results of these techniques revealed that there is a wide diversity of microbiota inhabiting the respiratory system. This diversity of microbiota is high in young CF patients who have better lung functions and subsequently need fewer courses of antibiotics and vice versa in the case of adults. The most dominant microbiota in infected lungs of CF patients are *P. aeruginosa*, BCC, and *A. xylosoxidans* [46].

3. Immune response in CF lung disease

Destruction of the respiratory airways may carry out due to the chronic CF infections. This damage is mediated by abnormal response of the host to airway infections, which in turn leads to irreversible bronchiectasis and lung function decline [47]. Many studies report that, bacterial infection and inflammation are leading to triggering of neutrophils [48]. Moreover, the dysfunction of CF-CFTR is a main cause of altered immune defense and disorders in the airway's environment. Appearance of neutrophil elastase (NE) is a good biomarker of disease [49].

The mutant CFTR gene leads to production of an abnormal protein, resulting in abnormal transport of salt and water across lining cells of the respiratory system, digestive system, and genital tracts. Insufficient water transport to the lining cells of the airways leads to formation of more thick and viscous respiratory secretions which clog small airways. Due to water reduction, the mucus becomes stagnant and infected with bacteria such as *P. aeruginosa* that may be inhaled or brought into the lungs through the mouth. Due to stagnant mucus, infection and chronic inflammation are developed. The tenacity of stagnant mucus is increased because the inflammatory cells are trapped in it. Due to accumulation of stagnant and infected mucus inside the airways, the bronchi dilate, and subsequently their walls are weakened. This phenomenon is called bronchiectasis that results in further airflow obstruction. According to the previous case, the respiratory cycle can be called the viscous cycle in which airway obstruction, inflammation, and infection are present, which lead to decrease of lung functions, respiratory failure, and death. Decrease of lung functions especially in children can also be due to exposure to smoking and polluted air, which also leads to pulmonary exacerbations.

The defective CF gene leads to defective CFTR and thick viscous secretions, which in turn lead to bronchial obstruction then to an infection then inflammation and finally bronchiectasis. Infection, inflammation, and bronchiectasis can lead to bronchial obstruction (**Figure 1**). Infection amplifies defective CF gene, which in turn leads to defective CFTR, which activates the resident airway inflammatory cells, which stimulate neutrophils and neutrophil products such as neutrophil elastase and monocytes, and finally bronchiectasis occurs (**Figure 2**).

The surface of epithelial lining cells of respiratory airways is dehydrated and acidified due to CFTR dysfunction, and abnormal mucociliary clearance is carried

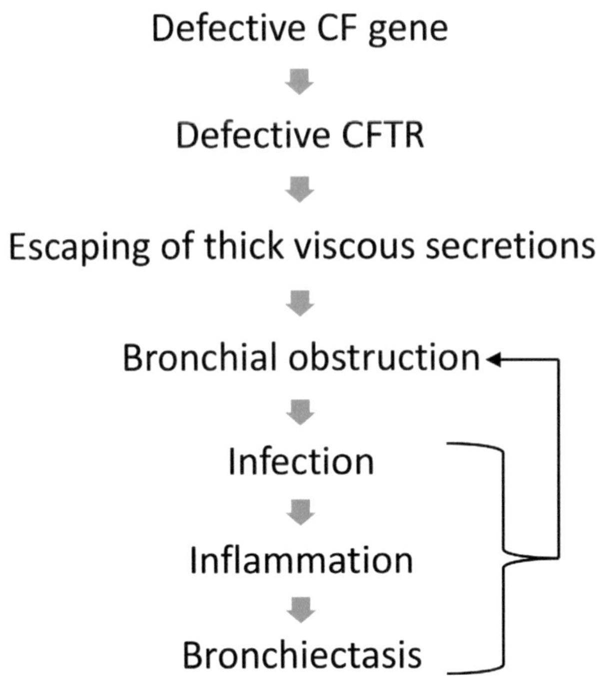

Figure 1.
Traditional pathophysiology of CF lung disease.

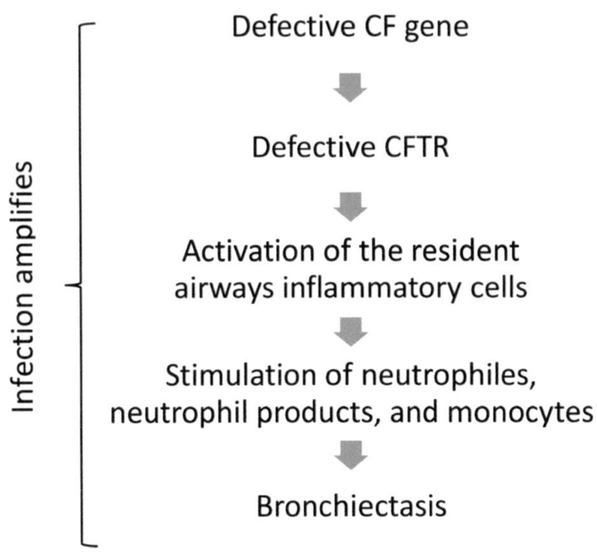

Figure 2.
Potential alternative mechanism for airway inflammation in CF lung disease.

out. Dehydration is carried out due to water loss, while acidification is carried out due to bicarbonate loss [50, 51]. The neutrophilic inflammatory response is higher in CF than in non-CF patients. However, the neutrophilic inflammatory response is reduced in neutrophil apoptosis. Neutrophils and their products are accumulated due to deficiency in mucociliary clearance and macrophage dysfunction [52]. The passage airways may destruct by the action of anti-proteases, such as alpha-1-antitrypsin, a serine protease inhibitor, and secretory leukocyte protease inhibitor. So, neutrophil products such as proteases and elastases are released to react with anti-proteases and therefore avoid their deleterious action toward the passage airways [53, 54].

Some substances act as mediators of immune response and serve as important biomarkers of disease progression, such as neutrophil elastase, which is abundant in induced sputum in children with CF compared to control children [55]. High level of neutrophil elastase in induced sputum indicates lung dysfunctions and bronchiectasis [13]. The inflammation of the passage airways in sputum is reduced after detection and using of effective antibiotics for treatment of a CF-pulmonary diseases [56]. Inflammatory proteins are considered potential biomarkers of disease in CF. For example, the blood plasma proteins are biomarkers of CF disease [57].

The common example of immune response in CF lung disease is the immune response to *P. aeruginosa* [58]. CFTR dysfunction predisposes the host to infection with *P. aeruginosa* and then allows for chronic infection and subsequent reduced opportunity for eradication. Moreover, *P. aeruginosa* interacts with other bacterial pathogens including *S. aureus* and *B. cepacia* complex to alter the inflammatory response [59].

4. Anti-inflammatory therapy of CF

4.1 Ibuprofen

Ibuprofen inhibits neutrophil migration and aggregation [60]. It improves the lung functions especially in patients younger than 13 years. Gastrointestinal bleeding may be associated with chronic therapy. Recent studies report that high-dose ibuprofen could slow the progression of lung disease in CF, particularly in children with mild disease [61]. Despite the efficacy of ibuprofen for CF lung disease therapy, its use is uncommon compared to other CF therapies due to severe adverse effects such as kidney failure and gastric bleeding [62].

4.2 Azithromycin

Azithromycin is a broad-spectrum antibiotic belonging to macrolide group, and at the same time, it has immunomodulatory effects, so it has high effectiveness in the treatment of CF lung disease and other chronic inflammatory conditions [63]. Azithromycin may be used for a very long period (chronic azithromycin) either with or without chronic *P. aeruginosa* infection [64]. With chronic *P. aeruginosa* infection, azithromycin is taken thrice weekly for 6 months to improve forced expiratory volume (FEV) and subsequently decrease the risk of pulmonary exacerbations. On the other hand, without chronic *P. aeruginosa* infection, azithromycin could reduce 50% of pulmonary exacerbations and improve weight, but without improvement of lung functions [65]. Azithromycin is recommended for CF treatment in patients suffering from chronic *P. aeruginosa* infection and those without chronic infection aged 6 years and older [66]. Despite the high durability of azithromycin, resistant bacteria are emerging, so the treatment should be reassessed every 6–12 months. Azithromycin is prohibited for patients with nontuberculous mycobacteria (NTM) unless it is prescribed in combination with other anti-mycobacterial medications as part of NTM therapy.

4.3 Corticosteroids and leukotriene receptor antagonists

Corticosteroids, especially its systemic forms, or cortisones are powerful anti-inflammatory agents which are widely used in the treatment of CF. Although systemic corticosteroids can intensively improve lung functions, they have adverse effects that outweigh any benefit [67]. Inhaled corticosteroids do not have any efficacy in the treatment of CF [68]. Therefore, the treatment of CF by systemic or inhaled corticosteroids is not recommended by the Cystic Fibrosis (CF) Foundation [66]. On the other hand, leukotriene receptor antagonists (LTRAs) are nonsteroidal oral medications, which are used as anti-inflammatory bronchoconstriction preventors. LTRAs block a chemical reaction that leads to inflammation in the airways. LTRAs are effective as antihistamines, and they are better than placebo, but less effective than nasal corticosteroids in improving symptoms and quality of life in patients with seasonal allergic rhinitis [69].

5. Treatment management of CF

CF carrier testing is recommended for everybody especially for Caucasian women whether they are considering pregnancy or already pregnant. CF-carrier test must be made before marriage, because the marriage of the positive CF-carriers leads offspring affected with CF, and vice versa. So, the early diagnosis of CF either before birth or for newborns allows for earlier and faster treatment in CF centers and avoidance of serious complications including poor growth. CF centers must be accredited by the CF Foundation. CF centers have multidisciplinary teams of physicians, nurses, respiratory therapists, dietitians, and social workers who can care for both adult and pediatric patients [70]. Good nutrition for affected persons with CF increases lung functions and life expectancy. Once CF disease is diagnosed, the patient must follow a nutrition program that is including a high-calorie diet, pancreatic enzymes and a liberal-fat. Essential vitamins must be supplemented to reduce the risk of deficiency of certain fat-soluble vitamins.

Although ill infants and young children with CF have intermittent cough and wheezing, structural and functional abnormalities in the lung as early as the first few months of life are detected. CF treatments include physical methods to eliminate thick secretions from the chest. CF treatments with chemical methods include prescription of different medications, such as dornase alfa and hypertonic saline as thinners of sticky airway secretions, albuterol as bronchodilator, tobramycin as inhaled antibiotic, and ibuprofen and azithromycin as anti-inflammatory drugs [71]. Preventive measures against CF or its complications necessarily require frequent follow-up for nutrition, lung functions, and screening for complications in an accredited CF center.

6. Conclusion

CF lung disease is one of the many causes of morbidity and mortality worldwide. CF lung disease has indefinite symptoms including airway obstruction, infection, and inflammation. This disease is associated with different microorganisms such as *P. aeruginosa*, *S. aureus*, and *B. cepacia* complex. Several medications are used as antimicrobial treatment for these pathogens. The airway microbiota is influenced by several factors including the environment, host, disease progression, and antibiotic treatment. Immune response to microbes in the CF airways is high due to dysfunction of CFTR protein. Although the recent therapies for airway infections and immune-inflammatory response are effective, they cannot fully stop disease progression. Today, CF lung disease has less risk because anti-inflammatory and antimicrobial therapies are in continuous development. Eventually, the authors recommend that, CF-carrier test must be made in particular before the marriage, early treatment of respiratory diseases especially if CF disease is diagnosed, avoidance of relatives marriage because it enhances an emergence of genetic diseases including CF, and finally, the treatment with corticosteroids (cortisone) must be under full control by a physician due to its severe adverse effects.

Acknowledgements

Authors sincerely thank National Organization for Drug Control and Research (NODCAR), Egypt, and Faculty of Science and Humanities, Shaqra University, Saudi Arabia for their support. Authors thank everybody aids in the introducing of this work as best as possible.

Conflict of interest

The authors declare no conflict of interest.

Notes

This chapter is concerned with CF-pulmonary diseases rather than other diseases of CF, because it is more widespread around the world and a common cause of morbidity and mortality especially in Caucasian areas as reported by the WHO.

Author details

Waleed Mohamed Abdulkhair[1]* and Mousa Abdullah Alghuthaymi[2]

1 General Department of Basic Medical Sciences, Microbiology Department, National Organization for Drug Control and Research (NODCAR), Giza, Egypt

2 Biology Department, Science and Humanities College, Shaqra University, Shaqra, Saudi Arabia

*Address all correspondence to: waleed_hamada@yahoo.com

References

[1] Andersen D. Cystic fibrosis of the pancreas and its relation to celiac disease: A clinical and pathological study. The American Journal of Diseases of Children. 1938;**56**:344-399. DOI: 10.1001/archpedi.1938.01980140114013

[2] Di Sant'agnese PEA, Andersen DH. Celiac syndrome; chemotherapy in infections of the respiratory tract associated with cystic fibrosis of the pancreas; observations with penicillin and drugs of the sulfonamide group, with special reference to penicillin aerosol. American Journal of Diseases of Children. 1946;**72**:17-61

[3] Lyczak JB, Cannon CL, Pier GB. Lung infections associated with cystic fibrosis. Clinical Microbiology Reviews. 2002;**15**:194-222. DOI: 10.1128/cmr.15.2.194-222.2002

[4] Khan TZ, Wagener JS, Bost T, Martinez J, Accurso FJ, Riches DW. Early pulmonary inflammation in infants with cystic fibrosis. American Journal of Respiratory and Critical Care Medicine. 1995;**151**:1075-1082. DOI: 10.1164/ajrccm/151.4.1075

[5] O'Sullivan BP, Freedman SD. Cystic fibrosis. Lancet. 2009;**373**:1891-1904. DOI: 10.1016/S0140-6736(09)60327-5

[6] Ouyang L, Grosse SD, Amendah DD, Schechter MS. Healthcare expenditures for privately insured people with cystic fibrosis. Pediatric Pulmonology. 2009;**44**:989-996. DOI: 10.1002/ppul.21090

[7] Walaa AS, Dina AM, Mona ME. Mutation spectrum of Egyptian children with cystic fibrosis. Springerplus. 2016;**5**(686):1-6. DOI: 10.1186/s40064-016-2338-7

[8] Saiman L, Siegel JD, LiPuma JJ, Brown RF, Bryson EA, Chambers MJ, et al. Infection prevention and control guideline for cystic fibrosis: 2013 update. Infection Control and Hospital Epidemiology. 2014;**35**(Suppl 1):S1-S67. DOI: 10.1086/676882

[9] Worlitzsch D, Tarran R, Ulrich M, Schwab U, Cekici A, Meyer KC, et al. Effects of reduced mucus oxygen concentration in airway *Pseudomonas* infections of cystic fibrosis patients. The Journal of Clinical Investigation. 2002;**109**:317-325. DOI: 10.1172/JCI13870

[10] Singh PK, Schaefer AL, Parsek MR, Moninger TO, Welsh MJ, Greenberg EP. Quorum-sensing signals indicate that cystic fibrosis lungs are infected with bacterial biofilms. Nature. 2000;**407**:762-764. DOI: 10.1038/35037627

[11] Sagel SD, Ronald LG, Julia E, Sharon M, Jane LB, Jeffrey SW, et al. Impact of *Pseudomonas* and *Staphylococcus* infection on inflammation and clinical status in young children with cystic fibrosis. The Journal of Pediatrics. 2009;**154**:183-188. DOI: 10.1016/j.jpeds.2008.08.001

[12] Gangell C, Gard S, Douglas T, Park J, de Klerk N, Keil T, et al. Inflammatory responses to individual microorganisms in the lungs of children with cystic fibrosis. Clinical Infectious Diseases. 2011;**53**:425-432. DOI: 10.1093/cid/cir399

[13] Pillarisetti N, Williamson E, Linnane B, Skoric B, Robertson CF, Robinson P, et al. Infection, inflammation, and lung function decline in infants with cystic fibrosis. American Journal of Respiratory and Critical Care Medicine. 2011;**184**:75-81. DOI: 10.1164/rccm.201011-1892OC

[14] Cogen J, Emerson J, Sanders DB, Ren C, Schechter MS, Gibson RL, et al.

Risk factors for lung function decline in a large cohort of young cystic fibrosis patients. Pediatric Pulmonology. 2015;**50**:763-770. DOI: 10.1002/ppul.23217

[15] Hudson VL, Wielinski CL, Regelmann WE. Prognostic implications of initial oropharyngeal bacterial flora in patients with cystic fibrosis diagnosed before the age of two years. The Journal of Pediatrics. 1993;**122**:854-860. DOI: 10.1016/S0022-3476(09)90007-5

[16] Mayer-Hamblett N, Aitken ML, Accurso FJ, Kronmal RA, Konstan MW, Burns JL, et al. Association between pulmonary function and sputum biomarkers in cystic fibrosis. American Journal of Respiratory and Critical Care Medicine. 2007;**175**:822-828. DOI: 10.1164/rccm.200609-1354OC

[17] Ahlgren HG, Andrea B, Jennifer SL, Joanie B, Elias M, Danuta R, et al. Clinical outcomes associated with *Staphylococcus aureus* and *Pseudomonas aeruginosa* airway infections in adult cystic fibrosis patients. BMC Pulmonary Medicine. 2015;**15**:67. DOI: 10.1186/s12890-015-0062-7

[18] Goss CH, Muhlebach MS. Review: *Staphylococcus aureus* and MRSA in cystic fibrosis. Journal of Cystic Fibrosis. 2011;**10**:298-306. DOI: 10.1016/j.jcf.2011.06.002

[19] Hoffman LR, Déziel E, D'Argenio DA, Lépine F, Emerson J, McNamara S, et al. Selection for *Staphylococcus aureus* small-colony variants due to growth in the presence of *Pseudomonas aeruginosa*. Proceedings of the National Academy of Sciences of the United States of America. 2006;**103**:19890-19895. DOI: 10.1073/pnas.0606756104

[20] Ren CL, Morgan WJ, Konstan MW, Schechter MS, Wagener JS, Fisher KA, et al. Presence of methicillin resistant *Staphylococcus aureus* in respiratory cultures from cystic fibrosis patients is associated with lower lung function. Pediatric Pulmonology. 2007;**42**:513-518. DOI: 10.1002/ppul.20604

[21] Sawicki GS, Rasouliyan L, Pasta DJ, Regelmann WE, Wagener JS, Waltz DA, et al. The impact of incident methicillin resistant *Staphylococcus aureus* detection on pulmonary function in cystic fibrosis. Pediatric Pulmonology. 2008;**43**:1117-1123. DOI: 10.1002/ppul.20914

[22] Muhlebach MS, Sonya LH, Elena BP, Melissa BM, Valeria T, Margaret K, et al. Multicenter observational study on factors and outcomes associated with different MRSA types in children with cystic fibrosis. Annals of the American Thoracic Society. 2015;**12**:864-871. DOI: 10.1513/AnnalsATS.201412-596OC

[23] Dasenbrook EC, Merlo CA, Diener-West M, Lechtzin N, Boyle MP. Persistent methicillin-resistant *Staphylococcus aureus* and rate of FEV decline in cystic fibrosis. American Journal of Respiratory and Critical Care Medicine. 2008;**178**:814-821. DOI: 10.1164/rccm.200802-327OC

[24] Sanders DB, Bittner RC, Rosenfeld M, Hoffman LR, Redding GJ, Goss CH. Failure to recover to baseline pulmonary function after cystic fibrosis pulmonary exacerbation. American Journal of Respiratory and Critical Care Medicine. 2010;**182**:627-632. DOI: 10.1164/rccm.200909-1421OC

[25] Dasenbrook EC, Checkley W, Merlo CA, Konstan MW, Lechtzin N, Boyle MP. Association between respiratory tract methicillin-resistant *Staphylococcus aureus* and survival in cystic fibrosis. Journal of the American Medical Association. 2010;**303**:2386-2392. DOI: 10.1001/jama.2010.791

[26] Smyth AR, Walters S. Prophylactic anti-staphylococcal antibiotics for

cystic fibrosis. Cochrane Database of Systematic Reviews. 2014;**11**:CD001912. DOI: 10.1002/14651858.CD001912.pub2

[27] Lo DKH, Hurley MN, Muhlebach MS, Smyth AR. Interventions for the eradication of methicillin-resistant *Staphylococcus aureus* (MRSA) in people with cystic fibrosis. Cochrane Database of Systematic Reviews. 2015;**2**:CD009650. DOI: 10.1002/14651858.CD009650.pub2

[28] Gilligan PH. Microbiology of airway disease in patients with cystic fibrosis. Clinical Microbiology Reviews. 1991;**4**:35-51. DOI: 10.1128/cmr.4.1.35

[29] Langton-Hewer SC, Smyth AR. Antibiotic strategies for eradicating *Pseudomonas aeruginosa* in people with cystic fibrosis. Cochrane Database of Systematic Reviews. 2009;**7**:CD004197. DOI: 10.1002/14651858.CD004197.pub3

[30] Regelmann WE, Elliott GR, Warwick WJ, Clawson CC. Reduction of sputum *Pseudomonas aeruginosa* density by antibiotics improves lung function in cystic fibrosis more than do bronchodilators and chest physiotherapy alone. The American Review of Respiratory Disease. 1990;**141**:914-921. DOI: 10.1164/ajrccm/141.4_Pt_1.914

[31] Mayer-Hamblett N, Kloster M, Rosenfeld M, Gibson RL, Retsch-Bogart GZ, Emerson J, et al. Impact of sustained eradication of new *Pseudomonas aeruginosa* infection on long-term outcomes in cystic fibrosis. Clinical Infectious Diseases. 2015;**61**:707-715. DOI: 10.1093/cid/civ377

[32] Mayer-Hamblett N, Rosenfeld M, Gibson RL, Ramsey BW, Kulasekara HD, Retsch-Bogart GZ, et al. *Pseudomonas aeruginosa in vitro* phenotypes distinguish cystic fibrosis infection stages and outcomes. American Journal of Respiratory and Critical Care Medicine. 2014;**190**:289-297. DOI: 10.1164/rccm.201404-0681OC

[33] Li Z, Kosorok MR, Farrell PM, Laxova A, West SE, Green CG, et al. Longitudinal development of mucoid *Pseudomonas aeruginosa* infection and lung disease progression in children with cystic fibrosis. Journal of the American Medical Association. 2005;**293**:581-588. DOI: 10.1001/jama.293.5.581

[34] Oliver A, Mulet X, Lõpez-Causapé C, Juan C. The increasing threat of *Pseudomonas aeruginosa* high-risk clones. Drug Resistance Updates. 2015;**22**:41-59. DOI: 10.1016/j.drup.2015.08.002

[35] Mogayzel PJ, Naureckas ET, Robinson KA, Brady C, Guill M, Lahiri T, et al. Cystic fibrosis foundation pulmonary guideline. Pharmacologic approaches to prevention and eradication of initial *Pseudomonas aeruginosa* infection. Annals of the American Thoracic Society. 2014;**11**:1640-1650. DOI: 10.1513/AnnalsATS.201404-166OC

[36] Merlo CA, Boyle MP, Diener-West M, Marshall BC, Goss CH, Lechtzin N. Incidence and risk factors for multiple antibiotic-resistant *Pseudomonas aeruginosa* in cystic fibrosis. Chest. 2007;**132**:562-568. DOI: 10.1378/chest.06-2888

[37] Zlosnik JEA, Zhou G, Brant R, Henry DA, Hird TJ, Mahenthiralingam E, et al. *Burkholderia* species infections in patients with cystic fibrosis in British Columbia, Canada. 30 years' experience. Annals of the American Thoracic Society. 2015;**12**:70-78. DOI: 10.1513/AnnalsATS.201408-395OC

[38] Lipuma JJ. Update on the *Burkholderia cepacia* complex. Current Opinion in Pulmonary Medicine.

2005;**11**:528-533. DOI: 10.1097/01.mcp.0000181475.85187.ed

[39] Horsley A, Webb K, Bright-Thomas R, Govan J, Jones A. Can early *Burkholderia cepacia* complex infection in cystic fibrosis be eradicated with antibiotic therapy? Frontiers in Cellular and Infection Microbiology. 2011;**1**:18. DOI: 10.3389/fcimb.2011.00018

[40] Regan KH, Bhatt J. Eradication therapy for *Burkholderia cepacia* complex in people with cystic fibrosis. Cochrane Database of Systematic Reviews. 2014;**24**:CD009876. DOI: 10.1002/14651858.CD009876.pub2

[41] Avgeri SG, Matthaiou DK, Dimopoulos G, Grammatikos AP, Falagas ME. Therapeutic options for *Burkholderia cepacia* infections beyond co-trimoxazole: A systematic review of the clinical evidence. International Journal of Antimicrobial Agents. 2009;**33**:394-404. DOI: 10.1016/j.ijantimicag.2008.09.010

[42] Parkins MD, Floto RA. Emerging bacterial pathogens and changing concepts of bacterial pathogenesis in cystic fibrosis. Journal of Cystic Fibrosis. 2015;**14**:293-304. DOI: 10.1016/j.jcf.2015.03.012

[43] Lipuma JJ. The changing microbial epidemiology in cystic fibrosis. Clinical Microbiology Reviews. 2010;**23**:299-323. DOI: 10.1128/CMR.00068-09

[44] Chmiel JF, Aksamit TR, Chotirmall SH, Dasenbrook EC, Elborn JS, LiPuma JJ, et al. Antibiotic management of lung infections in cystic fibrosis. I. the microbiome, methicillin-resistant *Staphylococcus aureus*, gram-negative bacteria, and multiple infections. Annals of the American Thoracic Society. 2014;**11**:1120-1129. DOI: 10.1513/AnnalsATS.201402-050AS

[45] Chmiel JF, Aksamit TR, Chotirmall SH, Dasenbrook EC, Elborn JS, LiPuma JJ, et al. Antibiotic management of lung infections in cystic fibrosis. II. Nontuberculous mycobacteria, anaerobic bacteria, and fungi. Annals of the American Thoracic Society. 2014;**11**:1298-1306. DOI: 10.1513/AnnalsATS.201405-203AS

[46] Caverly LJ, Zhao J, LiPuma JJ. Cystic fibrosis lung microbiome: Opportunities to reconsider management of airway infection: Cystic fibrosis lung microbiome. Pediatric Pulmonology. 2015;**50**:S31-S38. DOI: 10.1002/ppul.23243

[47] Gibson RL, Burns JL, Ramsey BW. Pathophysiology and management of pulmonary infections in cystic fibrosis. American Journal of Respiratory and Critical Care Medicine. 2003;**168**:918-951. DOI: 10.1164/rccm.200304-505SO

[48] Muhlebach MS, Stewart PW, Leigh MW, Noah TL. Quantitation of inflammatory responses to bacteria in young cystic fibrosis and control patients. American Journal of Respiratory and Critical Care Medicine. 1999;**160**:186-191. DOI: 10.1164/ajrccm.160.1.9808096

[49] Noah TL, Black HR, Cheng PW, Wood RE, Leigh MW. Nasal and bronchoalveolar lavage fluid cytokines in early cystic fibrosis. The Journal of Infectious Diseases. 1997;**175**:638-647. DOI: 10.1093/infdis/175.3.638

[50] Boucher RC. Airway surface dehydration in cystic fibrosis: Pathogenesis and therapy. Annual Review of Medicine. 2007;**58**:157-170. DOI: 10.1146/annurev.med.58.071905.105316

[51] Pezzulo AA, Tang XX, Hoegger MJ, Abou Alaiwa MH, Ramachandran S, Moninger TO, et al. Reduced airway surface pH impairs bacterial killing in the porcine cystic fibrosis lung. Nature. 2012;**487**:109-113. DOI: 10.1038/nature11130

[52] Alexis NE, Muhlebach MS, Peden DB, Noah TL. Attenuation of host defense function of lung phagocytes in young cystic fibrosis patients. Journal of Cystic Fibrosis. 2006;**5**:17-25. DOI: 10.1016/j.jcf.2005.11.001

[53] Birrer P, McElvaney NG, Rüdeberg A, Sommer CW, Liechti-Gallati S, Kraemer R, et al. Protease-antiprotease imbalance in the lungs of children with cystic fibrosis. American Journal of Respiratory and Critical Care Medicine. 1994;**150**:207-213. DOI: 10.1164/ajrccm.150.1.7912987

[54] Weldon S, McNally P, McElvaney NG, Elborn JS, McAuley DF, Wartelle J, et al. Decreased levels of secretory leucoprotease inhibitor in the *Pseudomonas*-infected cystic fibrosis lung are due to neutrophil elastase degradation. Journal of Immunology. 2009;**183**:8148-8156. DOI: 10.4049/jimmunol.0901716

[55] Sagel SD, Kapsner R, Osberg I, Sontag MK, Accurso FJ. Airway inflammation in children with cystic fibrosis and healthy children assessed by sputum induction. American Journal of Respiratory and Critical Care Medicine. 2001;**164**:1425-1431. DOI: 10.1164/rccm2104075

[56] Ordonez CL, Henig NR, Mayer-Hamblett N, Accurso FJ, Burns JL, Chmiel JF, et al. Inflammatory and microbiologic markers in induced sputum after intravenous antibiotics in cystic fibrosis. American Journal of Respiratory and Critical Care Medicine. 2003;**168**:1471-1475. DOI: 10.1164/rccm.200306-731OC

[57] Sagel SD, Thompson V, Chmiel JF, Montgomery GS, Nasr SZ, Perkett E, et al. Effect of treatment of cystic fibrosis pulmonary exacerbations on systemic inflammation. Annals of the American Thoracic Society. 2015;**12**:708-717. DOI: 10.1513/AnnalsATS.201410-493OC

[58] Lovewell RR, Patankar YR, Berwin B. Mechanisms of phagocytosis and host clearance of *Pseudomonas aeruginosa*. American Journal of Physiology. Lung Cellular and Molecular Physiology. 2014;**306**:L591-L603. DOI: 10.1152/ajplung.00335.2013

[59] Chattoraj SS, Murthy R, Ganesan S, Goldberg JB, Zhao Y, Hershenson MB, et al. *Pseudomonas aeruginosa* alginate promotes *Burkholderia cenocepacia* persistence in cystic fibrosis transmembrane conductance regulator knockout mice. Infection and Immunity. 2010;**78**:984-993. DOI: 10.1128/IAI.01192-09

[60] Konstan MW, Vargo KM, Davis PB. Ibuprofen attenuates the inflammatory response to *Pseudomonas aeruginosa* in a rat model of chronic pulmonary infection. Implications for antiinflammatory therapy in cystic fibrosis. The American Review of Respiratory Disease. 1990;**141**:186-192. DOI: 10.1164/ajrccm/141.1.186

[61] Lands LC, Stanojevic S. Oral non-steroidal anti-inflammatory drug therapy for lung disease in cystic fibrosis. Cochrane Database of Systematic Reviews. 2013;**6**:CD001505. DOI: 10.1002/14651858.CD001505.pub2

[62] Konstan MW, VanDevanter DR, Lawrence R, David JP, Ashley Y, Wayne JM, et al. Trends in the use of routine therapies in cystic fibrosis: 1995-2005. Pediatric Pulmonology. 2010;**45**:1167-1172. DOI: 10.1002/ppul.21315

[63] Zarogoulidis P, Papanas N, Kioumis I, Chatzaki E, Maltezos E, Zarogoulidis K. Macrolides: From *in vitro* anti-inflammatory and immunomodulatory properties to clinical practice in respiratory diseases. European Journal of Clinical Pharmacology. 2012;**68**:479-503. DOI: 10.1007/s00228-011-1161-x

[64] Saiman L, Marshall BC, Mayer-Hamblett N, Burns JL, Quittner AL, Cibene DA, et al. Azithromycin in patients with cystic fibrosis chronically infected with *Pseudomonas aeruginosa*: A randomized controlled trial. Journal of the American Medical Association. 2003;**290**:1749-1756. DOI: 10.1001/jama.290.13.1749

[65] Saiman L, Anstead M, Mayer-Hamblett N, Lands LC, Kloster M, Hocevar-Trnka J, et al. Effect of azithromycin on pulmonary function in patients with cystic fibrosis uninfected with *Pseudomonas aeruginosa*: A randomized controlled trial. Journal of the American Medical Association. 2010;**303**:1707-1715. DOI: 10.1001/jama.2010.563

[66] Mogayzel PJ, Edward TN, Karen AR, Gary M, Denis H, Jeffrey BH, et al. Cystic fibrosis pulmonary guidelines. Chronic medications for maintenance of lung health. American Journal of Respiratory and Critical Care Medicine. 2013;**187**:680-689. DOI: 10.1164/rccm.201207-1160OE

[67] Eigen H, Rosenstein BJ, FitzSimmons S, Schidlow DV. A multicenter study of alternate-day prednisone therapy in patients with cystic fibrosis. Cystic Fibrosis Foundation prednisone trial group. The Journal of Pediatrics. 1995;**126**:515-523. DOI: 10.1016/s0022-3476(95)70343-8

[68] Balfour-Lynn IM, Welch K. Inhaled corticosteroids for cystic fibrosis. Cochrane Database of Systematic Reviews. 2014;**10**:CD001915. DOI: 10.1002/14651858.CD001915.pub5

[69] Stelmach I, Korzeniewska A, Stelmach W, Majak P, Grzelewski T, Jerzynska J. Effects of montelukast treatment on clinical and inflammatory variables in patients with cystic fibrosis. Annals of Allergy, Asthma & Immunology. 2005;**95**:372-380. DOI: 10.1016/S1081-1206(10)61156-8

[70] Farrell PM, Rosenstein BJ, White TB, Accurso FJ, Castellani C, Cutting GR, et al. Guidelines for diagnosis of cystic fibrosis in newborns through older adults: Cystic Fibrosis Foundation consensus report. The Journal of Pediatrics. 2008;**153**:S4-S14. DOI: 10.1016/j.jpeds.2008.05.005

[71] Flume PA, O'Sullivan BP, Robinson KA, Goss CH, Mogayzel PJ Jr, Willey-Courand DB, et al. Cystic fibrosis pulmonary guidelines: Chronic medications for maintenance of lung health. American Journal of Respiratory and Critical Care Medicine. 2007;**176**:957-969. DOI: 10.1164/rccm.200705-664OC

Chapter 5

Lung Transplantation in Patients with Cystic Fibrosis

Prashant N. Mohite, Kavita Dave, Anna Reed and André R. Simon

Abstract

Cystic fibrosis (CF) is one of the most common indications for lung transplant (LTx) and nearly one-third of the LTx worldwide are performed in people with CF (PwCF). Due to vast developments in diagnostic modalities, antibiotic therapies, and management of associated comorbidities in dedicated and experienced centres, over the past few decades, more PwCF are reaching adulthood than ever before. This has increased the burden on transplant programs particularly in a universal donor shortage scenario. To improve the donor pool a diligent and proactive donor care management, acceptance of marginal organs and utilisation of ex-vivo lung perfusion systems for organ preservation, assessment, and improvement is being advocated widely. LTx is not a readily available therapy and the average waiting time is 18 months in the UK. Therefore, it is essential that PwCF are referred for LTx assessment when their disease is stable, before respiratory deterioration leads to overall deconditioning of the patients. Once listed for LTx, it is crucial to control waiting list mortality by prioritising rapidly deteriorating patients through schemes like the lung allocation score, national urgent and super-urgent waiting lists, and institutional highlighting of deteriorating patients that do not meet other urgent criteria. LTx in PwCF is challenging due to colonisation of the respiratory tract with multi-drug resistant organisms, associated comorbidities such as diabetes, liver disease, gastro-oesophageal reflux, and distal intestinal obstruction syndrome (DIOS) and CF-specific technical difficulties (adhesions due to prior pneumothoraces or pleurodesis, or bronchial collaterals that increase surgical time). Hilar lymphadenopathy and bronchial collaterals may increase surgical time, organ ischemia time, intra and post-operative bleeding, and blood transfusions. Advances in immunosuppression, prophylactic anti-viral and anti-fungal therapies, early ambulation and rigorous physiotherapy, and meticulous postoperative follow up with spirometry, x-rays, and bronchoscopies to detect rejection at the early stage followed by its efficient treatment have helped to improve post-LTx survival in the CF patients. Constant development in the surgical field with adoption of off-pump transplantation, sternal sparing bilateral thoracotomy approach, and utilisation of mechanical circulatory assist as a bridge to transplant and as a support for primary graft failure strives for better outcomes. However, chronic lung allograft dysfunction, chronic refractory infections, malignancies, and CF associated comorbidities remain major determinants of post-LTx long term survival. Despite this, CF patients are often good candidates for re-do LTx with improving survival outcomes. In this chapter, we are compiling the different aspects of LTx in PwCF emphasising the advances in bridge to transplantation, the surgical approach, management of primary graft failure, and immunosuppression as well as complications post-transplant.

Keywords: cystic fibrosis, lung transplantation, advances, minimally invasive lung transplantation, off pump lung transplantation

1. Introduction

While it took years following the first human LTx in 1963 for this procedure to become a gold standard therapy in the management of end-stage lung disease, the procedure took off in the 80s following the introduction of Cyclosporin in medical practice. The first transplant in a patient with CF was a heart-lung transplant performed by Magdi Yacoub in Harefield Hospital in the United Kingdom [1]. Since then, nearly ten thousand patients with CF have undergone LTx worldwide [2]. According to the 36th adult lung and heart-lung transplant report comprising more than 69000 adult LTx in the ISHLT registry, 15.2% of all adult LTx were performed in PwCF [2]. Although the number of transplants performed for each indication has increased ever since, the proportion of patients transplanted for CF continues to fall, now accounting for 13% of total adult lung transplants, compared with over 15% five years ago [2, 3]. With constant improvement in knowledge, better management of infective exacerbations, developments in the field of antimicrobials and breakthrough modulator therapy for PwCF, survival has improved in CF patients significantly [4–6]. However, this may have led not only to increasing numbers of PwCF meeting criteria for LTx but unfortunately, also to delayed referrals, referral of sicker patients with comorbidities, and patients with complex colonisations of multi-drug resistant organisms. Despite this, with 9.9 years of median survival and 12.4 years of conditional survival in patients that survive beyond the first year, PwCF demonstrate the best survival compared to any other indication for LTx [2]. Moreover, survival in ISHLT registry (1992 to 2017) stratified in 3 eras show a significant improvement in the survival of PwCF in the recent era when compared with other indications for LTx [2]. This is mainly due to the younger age and good other end-organ function of these patients at the time of transplantation. On the other hand, CF patients when compared to other indications for LTx pose a set of exclusive challenges. Familiarity, experience and expertise of the transplant team to deal with these problems make a significant difference in the outcomes.

2. Patient selection

2.1 Indications and contraindications of LTx in CF

With a scarcity of donor organs and higher mortality in LTx recipients compared to other organs, health economics would support offering a limited supply of donor organs to recipients expected to benefit the most. However, the onus to identify such recipients falls upon timely referral and listing of the candidates for potential LTx. A clinical window where the patient is symptomatic enough to require LTx but strong enough to survive the operative trauma varies with the individual patient. Generally, when the FEV1 in PwCF drops below 30%, their expected median survival is around 2 years [7]. However, FEV1 is not a reliable indicator of survival as many with CF with longstanding low lung function may survive without transplantation. Currently though, in the absence of a better option, it remains the best available indicator for referral and listing purposes. Inadequacy of clinical parameters to sufficiently predict survival in CF patients raise a need for mortality prediction models. One of the first such comprehensive models recognised age, respiratory microbiology, height, FEV1, annual number of hospital admissions and courses of home intravenous antibiotics as the most important predictors of 2-year mortality [8]. However, the authors also admit that their model is no better than the widely used FEV1 < 30% predicted. Thus, referral of patients for transplant based either on their model probability of dying within 2 years or on an FEV1 of less than 30% predicted could result in a high rate of premature referral, as a substantial proportion of patients predicted to die within 2 years based on these criteria would survive this period. Therefore, it is wise to take into consideration risk factors associated with early mortality in PwCF when shortlisting them for LTx. One of the biggest CF databases, the UK CF Registry reviewed records from 2005 to 2015 on 6181 individuals, and acknowledged strong associations of *Burkholderia cepacia* infection, CF-related diabetes, and more hospital days on IV antibiotics with decreasing survival [9]. A Canadian CF registry analysis identified older age at diagnosis, diabetes, and deteriorating FEV1 as predictors of reduced survival [10] whilst a recent meta-analysis based upon 11 studies identified *Burkholderia cenocepacia* and ascending chronological year of LTx as predictors of post-LTx mortality [11]. Referring physicians whilst focusing on the FEV1, should also pay special attention to these risk factors for poor survival when considering referral to a transplant centre.

Contraindications of LTx in the CF are similar to other end-stage lung disease causes and are broadly divided into absolute and relative contraindications. A consensus document for the selection of LTx candidates offers a thorough review into the contraindications for LTx (**Table 1**) [12].

2.2 Criteria for referral and listing

Early or sometimes premature referral of PwCF to transplant centres offers patients a chance of early transplant assessment to maximise their window of opportunity for donor offers and a LTx. Additionally, early referral has the potential to identify modifiable contraindications to LTx or risk factors of transplant mortality allowing these to be treated and optimised before requiring listing. A delayed referral carries a risk of insufficient time to wait and less number of donor offers to the referred patients. Candidates may miss their window of opportunity and be removed from the waiting list due to clinical deterioration or worse. An ideal time of listing any candidate for LTx is when the benefits from the procedure balance its risk. It is not unusual practice at transplant centres to send patients back to the referring physicians for not meeting the criteria of listing post-assessment but identifying them as future candidates. A 2006 ISHLT update for selection of transplant candidates for the first time separated referral and listing criteria emphasising a timely referral of the end-stage lung disease candidate to transplantation centres [13]. These were revised in a 2014 update as summarised in **Table 2** [14].

2.3 Pre-operative work-up

Transplant teams while assessing referred CF patients for LTx should ask two vital questions- (i) Is a transplant required- in other words, is the transplant going to improve survival and quality of life? (ii) Is the patient transplantable? – i.e. is the patient going to survive the transplant?

Transplant evaluation requires a medical assessment, psychological assessment, and in some countries, financial assessment. The medical assessment requires an admission for 2–3 days so that a patient can have multiple investigations and be reviewed by the multi-disciplinary team (MDT) (**Table 3**) [15]. Additional investigations that may be

Absolute contraindications	
History of malignancy with less than 5 years of disease free interval	
Untreatable significant dysfunction of another major organ system	
Coronary artery disease not amenable to revascularization	
Acute medical instability (sepsis, myocardial infarction, liver failure)	
Uncorrectable bleeding diathesis	
Chronic infection with highly virulent and/or resistant microbes	
Evidence of active *Mycobacterium tuberculosis* infection	
Significant chest wall or spinal deformity	
BMI $\geq$ 35.0 kg/m^2	
Current or history of non-adherence to medical therapy	
Psychologic conditions with inability to cooperate with medical team	
Absence of adequate or reliable social support system	
Severely limited functional status with poor rehabilitation potential	
Substance abuse or dependence	
Relative contraindications	
Age > 65 years in association with low physiologic reserve	
BMI 30.0–34.9 kg/m^2	
Progressive or severe malnutrition	
Severe, symptomatic osteoporosis	
Extensive prior chest surgery with lung resection	
Mechanical ventilation and/or extracorporeal life support	
Colonisation/infection with highly resistant or virulent organisms	
Infection with hepatitis B and/or C	
Infection with HIV	
Infection with Burkholderia cenocepacia, Burkholderia gladioli	
Infection with multi-drug–resistant Mycobacterium abscessus	
Atherosclerotic disease burden	
Diabetes mellitus, systemic hypertension, epilepsy	
Central venous obstruction, peptic ulcer disease, gastroesophageal reflux	

Table 1.
Absolute and relative contraindications for LTx in CF.

required include CT coronary angiogram (CTCA) in PwCF aged over 40 years or right heart catheterisation in severe pulmonary hypertension. All referrals require a dental assessment before listing, but PwCF may require assessment by ENT or gastroenterology doctors in addition. Psychology, palliative care and physiotherapy review during their assessment provides insight on a patient's suitability to undergo transplantation, and social support is also explored during this time. In some countries, financial evaluation is necessary to ensure a potential recipient can afford the immediate transplant care, lifelong aftercare and medications, and management of complications. Following this period of assessment, patients are subsequently discussed at MDT meetings, which include respiratory physicians, transplant surgeons, psychologists, immunologists, radiologists, dietitans and physiotherapists. After discussion, outcomes for each patient

Timing of referral
FEV1 < 30% pred or falling rapidly despite optimal therapy
A 6-minute walk distance <400 m
Pulmonary hypertension in absence of hypoxic exacerbation
Clinical decline- increasing exacerbations with -
(i) Acute resp. failure requiring NIV
(ii) Increasing antibiotic resistance and poor clinical recovery from exacerbations
(iii) Worsening nutritional status despite supplementation
(iv) Pneumothorax
(v) Life threatening hemoptysis despite bronchial embolization
Timing of listing
Chronic respiratory failure with hypoxia alone ($PaO2 < 8$ kPa)
Chronic respiratory failure with hypercapnia ($PaCO2 > 6.6$ kPa)
Long-term NIV
Pulmonary hypertension
Frequent hospitalisation
Rapid lung function decline
WHO Functional Class IV

Table 2.
Timing of referral and timing of listing for LTx in CF patients.

include decision for active listing, further information required, rejection as unsuitable, or deferral as too well.

2.4 Waiting list

The time spent by potential recipients on the LTx waiting list depends on various factors including blood group, HLA antibody status and the size of pleural cavities. Whilst on the waiting list, patients are encouraged to exercise regularly, achieve or maintain a healthy BMI, avoid frequent infective exacerbations, and inform any changes in circumstances urgently. Transplant coordinators maintain contact with patients on the waiting list, update records, educate patients and communicate between all members of the transplant team. Traditionally, organ offering systems take into account time spent on the waiting list and the clinical status of the candidates, but influenced by the urgency of transplantation. With this freedom of recipient selection to the transplant centres, fairness in the distribution of the donor organs to the most worthy recipients may be jeopardised. A study looking into 2213 lung-only registrations into the UK Transplant Registry between 2004 and 2014 showed discrepancies between the risk profile and probability of LTx. The chance of LTx after listing differed by the combined effect of disease category and centre, height (taller patients having a greater chance of transplant) and blood group (blood group 'O' having highest waiting mortality) [16].

The ideal recipient for any donor organ is the one with urgent need of transplantation along with the longest expected post-transplant survival. The Lung Allocation Score (LAS) system adopted in the US in 2005 incorporated estimated survival benefit offered by LTx by 1 year after surgery and medical urgency. Since its introduction, the number of deaths on the waiting list in the US has reduced

Blood tests
Full blood count, Coagulation studies, Blood glucose, Blood group
Kidney function, Liver function
Lipid profile, Thyroid function
HLA status, Panel reactive antibody status
Radiology studies
Chest CT, Sinus CT
Abdominal ultrasound
Functional studies
Lung function: Spirometry, lung volumes and diffusion
Arterial blood gases
6-min walk test
Cardiac: ECG, Echocardiogram, right heart catheterisation
Bone mineral density
Infection screen
Sputum m/c/s, fungi and mycobacteria
Mantoux test
Midstream urine
Swabs for MRSA
Serology for HIV, hepatitis B, hepatitis C
Serology for cytomegalovirus, Ebstein-Barr virus, Varicella zoster
Serology for Chlamydia pneumoniae
Malignancy screen
Sputum cytology
Papanicolau smear
Prostate specific antigen
Mammography
Faecal occult blood screening
Autoimmune screen
ANA, ENA, DNA antibody, Rheumatoid factor, ANCA, Immunoglobulins
Creatine kinase
Compliance screen Serum cotinine
Consultant referrals
Dental, Ear, nose and throat, Gastroenterology
Nutrition
Physiotherapy

Table 3.
Assessment for LTx in CF patients.

from 500/year to 300/year, the distribution of recipients has changed, and the number of LTx increased despite no substantial increase in organ donors with no decrease in 1-year survival after LTx, even though sicker patients were undergoing transplant [17]. With the introduction of the LAS, the number of LTx for PwCF increased by 25%, 70% of CF patients were transplanted within 1 year of being listed, and 1-year waiting-list mortality decreased from 15–10% [18]. The LAS was then adopted by Eurotransplant who distribute lungs between donor countries if they cannot be used within the donor's country of origin. After 3 years, the US results were imitated in Germany [19]. However, some reports have shown that the LAS increases the complexity of the post-transplant course and postoperative mortality [20, 21] and in some cases, reduced survival outcomes irrespective of risk profile [22]. Current allocation policy in the US initially utilises donor organ location and age to match with compatible wait-listed patients, followed by the LAS value, ABO blood type, thoracic cavity size and immunological compatibilities to ultimately select a match.

In the UK, between 2004 and 2014, 79.2% of patients with chronic obstructive pulmonary disease (COPD) received a transplant by 3 years of wait on the list versus 61.3% of PwCF and 48.9% of those with pulmonary fibrosis (PF). During the same period, patients with COPD had the lowest mortality on the list. In comparison, PwCF had a 230% higher chance of death on the list without LTx [16]. To optimise this disparity in organ allocation, in May 2017 the Cardiothoracic Advisory Group introduced an urgent and super-urgent lung allocation scheme in which patients at high risk of death without a LTx are prioritised at a national level [23]. In this scheme, patients supported with ECMO (extracorporeal membrane oxygenation) or iLA (interventional lung assist) as a bridge to transplant are prioritised on a national super-urgent waiting list, whilst severely unwell patients particularly in CF patient, worsening hypoxia and hypercapnia, persistently low pH, refractory right heart failure and ongoing massive hemoptysis can be recommended for the national urgent waiting list. Other policies in the UK include small adults (≥16 years of age and ≤ 155 cm of height) receiving offers of lungs from paediatric donors before other adults, (but after paediatric patients,) and priority is given to blood group identical recipients over blood group compatible recipients. In some cases, 'zonal centre' priority is given to patients at a centre if the donor is located within that centre's allocation zone [23]. However, the current system remain inefficient in prioritising patients depending upon the type of lung disease, and building individual risk profiles combining the factors such as urgency, height, and blood group. All current organ allocation systems strive to achieve the best post-transplant survival rates whilst reducing waiting list mortality, but remain far from ideal. Current systems should continue to undergo periodic evaluations, adopt practices from other systems, and remain dynamic to outcome-driven changes. The zonal allocation should depend on a distance rather than arbitrary geographical boundaries.

3. Lung transplantation

3.1 Donors

Availability of donor organs remains the most important limiting factor for transplantation as lungs, in particular, have the lowest harvest rate. The Eurotransplant registry reports utilisation of lungs from only 698 donors out of 1192 registrants in the year 2019 which is significantly lower compared to abdominal organs [24]. Significant progress has been made in the last decade to improve the donor pool for lungs, but there remains a huge scope for further development. Donation after circulatory death (DCD) is becoming commonplace with a recent review of ISHLT data showing comparable five-year survival in recipients receiving lungs from donors after brain death (DBD) against DCD (63% vs. 61%) [25].

Metanalyses comparing LTx outcomes dependent on the type of donation have shown no difference in survival, primary graft dysfunction (PGD) or acute rejection [26, 27]. Protocol-based management of multiorgan brain dead donors with a focus on lung donation in recent years have significantly improved lung utilisation rates [28]. A ventilation strategy with a low tidal volume and higher PEEP, along with a neutral or negative fluid balance helps protect potential donor lungs [29].

Standard lung donor criteria have been liberalised in the last two decades with an increasing proportion of marginal donor lungs being utilised for LTx with equivalent outcomes. A review of the UNOS database showed reduced 1-year survival with the use of marginal donor lungs, especially in high-risk recipients [30]; however, the survival of these patients on the waiting list without transplantation is questionable. Moreover, it's the high-risk recipients and not marginal donors that are associated with poor outcomes [31]. A lung donor score (LDS) based upon past medical history, smoking history, age, arterial blood gases, chest X-ray, and bronchoscopy findings, that accurately predicts the likelihood of organ acceptance and recipient mortality may facilitate donor risk assessment and patient selection [32]. Ex-vivo lung perfusion (EVLP) is now an established therapy to repair and evaluate marginal lungs for transplantation with comparable post-transplant outcomes [33–35].

To expand the donor pool, more countries are embracing an 'opt-out' system for organ donation. In Europe, the 2018 figures of lung donor utilisation rate were significantly higher in Austria and Belgium (9.8 and 10.8 ppm) where they have opt-out systems for organ donation, compared to Germany and the Netherlands (3.8 and 4.7 ppm) where an opt-in system remains [36]. The waiting list mortality rates in countries with high donation rates are lower compared to those in countries with low donation rates (7% vs. 12% at 1 year), with higher quality donor lungs more often used in these countries with high donation rates, thus offering a chance of better outcomes in recipients [37].

3.2 Challenges in LTx for CF

3.2.1 Preoperative procedures

The average annual incidence of pneumothorax in PwCF is 1:167 patients per year and 3.4% of CF patients will experience a pneumothorax during their lifetime [38]. According to current CF Foundation practice guidelines, a chest drain is recommended for large pneumothoraces or small pneumothoraces with clinical instability, whilst surgical pleurodesis is recommended for recurrent, large pneumothoraces [39]. The incidence of CF patients with a history of pleural intervention undergoing LTx is increasing as patients are being offered alternative interventional therapies before resorting to LTx.

The inflammatory/chronic infective component of CF independently contributes to increased pleural adhesions [40]. Dense pleural adhesions encountered during LTx in such patients increases surgical time, bleeding, blood transfusion requirement (that may further increase the chance of primary graft failure (PGD)), renal injury, prolonged respiratory wean and early mortality [41, 42]. Some groups, however, report no difference in operative outcomes despite pleural adhesions in PwCF [40, 43, 44]. It is worth noting that the LAS nor the ISHLT Registry consider previous cardiothoracic procedures as a contraindication to LTx.

In a multicentre study of CT scan scoring in PwCF based on infection/inflammation, air trapping/hypoperfusion, normal/hyperperfusion, and bulla/cysts, infection/inflammation was found to have a significant predictive value for survival [45]. Careful and detailed studies of CTs for pleural thickening, irregularity and calcification before listing for LTx is recommended to anticipate operative challenges and risk stratification. Avoidance of CPB, starting the procedure on the side of fewer adhesions, minimising blood loss by meticulous adhesiolysis and the presence of an experienced surgeon may prove helpful. PwCF may require lung resection for localised severe bronchiectasis, atelectasis, bronchopleural fistula refractory to medical management and severe hemoptysis refractory to conservative management [46, 47]. This not only causes pleural adhesions, but can also lead to loss of pleural cavity volume. At LTx evaluation, such patients require strategic planning while setting donor size parameters; they may require a donor lung reduction or lobar lung implantation.

3.2.2 Preop ECMO and mechanical ventilation

It is not uncommon for PwCF to suffer an infective exacerbation causing acute hypercapnic respiratory failure with worsening respiratory acidosis. Most exacerbations are managed with antibiotics and chest physiotherapy, but some require respiratory support with inhaled oxygen or escalation to non-invasive ventilation (NIV). Patients with deteriorating gas exchange despite NIV either require endotracheal intubation and invasive mechanical ventilation (IMV) or ECMO despite or to minimise IMV. Once an acceptable gas exchange is established with ECMO, sedation wean and extubation or tracheostomy should be performed in these patients to allow for ongoing physiotherapy rehabilitation.

Recent evidence from the UNOS database comprising 14,320 patients in the LAS era showed an association between pre-transplant ECMO and IMV with 30-day mortality as well as prolonged hospital length of stay after LTx [48, 49]. The Extracorporeal Life Support Organisation (ELSO) Registry showed 52% survival in CF patients supported on ECMO [50]. Fuehner et al. demonstrated improved survival in patients bridged to LTx with an "awake ECMO" strategy when compared with those managed with IMV (80% vs. 50% at 6 months), emphasising the potential advantages of minimising time sedated [51]. The key benefits of maintaining patients awake on ECMO is the avoidance of complications associated with sedation, intubation, IMV, and immobilisation. They can undertake active physiotherapy helping to reduce the rate of muscle wasting and preventing pressure sores. Patients are encouraged to eat and drink without enteral feed if possible. Meeting family and social media helps to maintain a positive mood, and suboptimal therapy or complications can be detected at an earlier stage as patients can identify and communicate symptoms of dizziness, breathlessness, and pain [52].

3.3 Procedure of LTx

Despite early success and advantages of heart-lung transplantation for CF (fewer anastomoses, shorter ischaemic times and re-utilisation of recipient's heart in a "domino" transplant), it has been superseded by LTx due to donor organ shortage and equivalent outcomes [53]. Bilateral sequential LTx in which unilateral pneumonectomy and donor lung implantation are performed in sequence is the standard operation for a suppurative disease like CF. However, single-LTx after synchronous or metachronous contralateral pneumonectomy for PwCF resulting in an asymmetric chest and lung volume mismatch may be an acceptable functional therapeutic option [54, 55].

The CF patient population consists of a large proportion of children and small adults that are not suitable recipients for most adult sized donors leading to an increase in the waiting list mortality. For a marginal size mismatch, peripheral lung resection, also known as 'lung shaving' may suffice, however, donor lung lobectomy to utilise only the upper or lower (preferred option) lobe dependent on the recipient pleural cavity size may be required [56, 57]. Bi-partitioning lobar LTx is a bilateral lobar transplant from a single donor lung. This can be performed to maximise the donor pool, but is not a popular procedure due to technical challenges [58]. Living-donor lobar LTx (LDLLT) is lifesaving in countries with low cadaveric donation and for patients deemed unable to await a cadaveric LTx [59]. Two lobes obtained from live donors can adequately support an adult CF patient and the morbidity from lobectomy to the healthy donor is minimal. A study where 84% of the cohort were CF patients undergoing LDLLT showed a survival of 70% and 45% at 1 and 5 years, which is comparable with double-lung cadaveric transplantation according to the ISHLT Registry (74% and 49.5% at 1 and 5 years) in in the same year [60].

3.4 Advances in LTx surgery

3.4.1 Minimally invasive LTx

For double LTx in CF, the clamshell is a conventional approach that offers a direct vision to the heart and lung hila, but can cause sternal dehiscence, malalignment, wound dehiscence and rarely mediastinitis. These complications are thought to be under-reported, but cause significant morbidity through readmissions, multiple surgical debridements and prolonged wound care. Infection can be difficult to treat in the presence of steroid-induced osteoporosis, breathing-induced mobility in healing sternal edges, and immunosuppression. Sternal sparing bilateral thoracotomy approach may be less painful and may support early extubation, ambulation, and rehabilitation [61]. This approach spares the internal mammary arteries, causing less blood loss, and is superior cosmetically to the clamshell incision. A requirement of long instruments and telescopic surgical skills for this approach is a myth. Utilisation of a modified rib spreader, with movable and adjustable blades provides optimum exposure without injuring the ribs. For emergency conversion to CPB, apart from peripheral access via the groin, one can cannulate via the thoracotomy.

3.4.2 Role of mechanical circulatory support in LTx surgery

Double LTx is conventionally performed with the aid of cardio-pulmonary bypass. As bilateral sequential LTx became commonplace, the use of CPB during the procedure declined. A comparative study of LTx in CF shows that the implantation of both lungs on CPB after bilateral pneumonectomy and airway decontamination does offer a protective effect against early graft infection [62]. CBP provides complete respiratory support and haemodynamic stability, ease of hilar dissection and retraction of the heart during the LTx, but can induce an inflammatory response, bleeding, (and thus increased requirement of blood transfusions), and a higher incidence of PGD [63]. Significantly lower survival was observed in CF patients undergoing LTx with the utilisation of extracorporeal circulation [64]. Off-pump surgery may avoid complications caused by circulatory support but is susceptible to periods of hypotension, hypothermia, and hypoxia. It also exposes the new lung to the entire cardiac output potentially causing acute lung injury and PGD.

Off-pump LTx may require emergency conversion to CPB in case of inability to tolerate single lung ventilation, hemodynamic instability, or uncontrolled bleeding. Off-pump LTx requiring emergent conversion to CPB is by default a part of the on-pump group in several reports comparing on-pump and off-pump procedures, which has found worse outcomes in the on-pump group [65, 66]. In the quest of a fair comparison, a further study segregated cases with unplanned CPB conversion and found that despite this segregation, patients with comparable preoperative demographic and risk profiles demonstrated better early postoperative outcomes including early survival with an off-pump strategy for LTx in comparison to an on-pump strategy. While a considerable proportion of high-risk patients require intraoperative conversion from off-pump to CPB with suboptimal outcomes, there is no significant benefit to employing an elective on-pump strategy in this high-risk group [67]. Although elective use of CPB for LTx has decreased in recent years, mechanical circulatory support of some form is still necessary during LTx in the presence of pulmonary hypertension, suboptimal cardiac function, severe respiratory disease, and marginal donor organs with an insufficient gas exchange when performing one-lung ventilation. Instead of CPB, ECMO that can potentially be continued post-operatively until the donor organs recover and pulmonary pressures alleviate is increasingly being utilised. ECMO offers cardiopulmonary support without cardiotomy suction, venous reservoir, a large amount of prime, and may avoid some complications associated with CPB. A meta-analysis of 7 studies comprising 785 patients comparing CPB and ECMO in LTx showed a lower rate of primary graft dysfunction, bleeding, renal failure requiring dialysis, tracheostomy, intraoperative transfusions, intubation time, and hospital stay along with a trend towards lower mortality in the ECMO group [68]. Elective use of mechanical circulatory support in LTx for CF is now limited to severe secondary pulmonary hypertension or if additional cardiac surgery is required, such as atrial septal defect closure. Optimisation with Milrinone and nitric oxide before a trial of pulmonary artery clamping can be helpful to assess if mechanical support may be required. If there is hemodynamic instability and inadequate gas exchange on single lung ventilation, the operation should continue under ECMO support, whilst emergency CPB can be ustilised in case of catastrophic bleeding, irreversible arrhythmia or hemodynamic instability.

3.4.3 Re-transplantation

CF patients often become candidates for re-transplantation due to their young age at the time of their primary transplant. PwCF have overall good post-transplant survival but also suffer a higher incidence of bronchiolitis obliterans syndrome (BOS). BOS, primary graft failure (PGD) and irreversible airway complications (stenosis and dehiscence) are the main causes for lung re-transplantation. Pseudomonal airway colonisation before and after LTx is thought to be associated with the increased prevalence of BOS in CF patients [69]. CF recipients are at higher risk of acute cellular rejection and subsequent BOS due to the enhanced immune activation associated with CF, their younger age and higher prevalence of donor specific antibodies [70, 71]. Scarcity of donor organs and suboptimal outcomes have always raised doubts about the validity and ethics of re-transplantation, especially as historically, the survival post-re-transplantation has remained inferior compared to the primary transplantation. Interestingly though, rates of BOS has shown an improved trend with 1-year survival increasing from 47% in the 1990s to 72–78% in the last 15 years [73–75]. Re-transplantation in non-ambulatory, ventilated patients, with PGD, anastomotic dehiscence, or less than a year since primary transplantation is associated with higher mortality [72–75]. Careful recipient selection with preoperative optimization in terms of nutrition and functional status, along with end-organ function are vital for successful re-transplantation.

4. Complications of LTx in CF

PwCF continue to demonstrate the best survival compared to other indications for LTx [76, 77], but suffer the same complications as those without CF to varying extents. Within the first month, primary graft dysfunction, acute infections, and technical complications dominate the cause for admissions, transitioning to also include rejection in the first year. Rejection and infection remain complicating factors throughout a recipient's life, with malignancy an increasing risk the longer a recipient remains on immunosuppression [77, 78].

4.1 PGD

Primary graft dysfunction (PGD) is the main cause of death within the first 30 days post-operatively [78], and is a form of acute lung injury that involves a wide spectrum of signs and symptoms within the first 72 hours of transplantation. For this reason, it is also known as the "re-implantation response". PGD is the consequence of an inflammatory response triggered by injury to the donor, graft or recipient, ischaemia, and reperfusion, and can cause a decrease in oxygenation with minimal pulmonary infiltrates caused by oedema, through to complete graft failure and death or re-transplantation. PGD is caused by the activation of pulmonary macrophages and circulating leukocytes and is divided into two phases – a first acute phase of lung schaemia and reperfusion injury, which drives the second phase mediated by massive neutrophil recruitment which amplifies the initial innate immune reaction.

A number of risk factors for development of PGD have been identified; in general, donor factors tend to impact the initial 24 hours post-transplantation, whilst the recipient factors affect later outcomes. Donor-related risk factors include sex, age, smoking history, ischaemic time, and brain-death-associated lung injury [79, 80]. Given the underlying pathophysiology of PGD, the approach to management is based on the treatment of ARDS (acute respiratory distress syndrome) using protective IMV and maintaining a negative fluid balance. However, this treatment plan is complicated by patients who may not tolerate permissive hypercapnia cardiologically, and fragile renal function due to multiple insults in the operative and immediate post-operative period.

It has been shown that lung recipients who develop PGD have a marked graft and systemic inflammatory response, and that the timing and grade of PGD severity has implications to the risk of developing BOS (bronchiolitis obliterans) later [81, 82].

4.2 Infections

Post-transplant infections remain a significant source of morbidity and mortality in all recipients, but this is complicated by the nature of the multi-resistant organisms found in CF recipients due to repeated antibiotic courses. It has long been accepted that PwCF are chronically colonised with bacteria, and so finding positive microbiology in the sputum of transplanted PwCF does not necessitate an acute infection, but equally, transplanting the lungs does not eradicate individuals with CF of the bacteria which remain colonised in the upper airways and the sinuses. PwCF colonised with *Mycobacterium abscessus* or *Bulkholderia cenocepacia* cannot be transplanted in most centres due to the high morbidity and mortality rates associated with these conditions post-transplantation. Though there have been some success in transplanting PwCF who have negative sputum for *M. abscessus* pre-transplantation but remain on treatment [83–85].

It is just as important to consider the donor's microbiological profile. All donors are screened for obvious reasons for HIV, hepatitis B and hepatitis C, but where donors have died from undiagnosed infections, the risk of transmitting a potentially lethal infection into a recipient has to be considered. In addition, the longer a potential donor is ventilated, the more likely they are to become colonised with antibiotic-resistant flora, complicating a future transplant. BAL before harvesting or implantation is useful to culture and therefore guide antibiotic management in the peri-operative and immediate post-operative period.

Like any major surgery, surgical site infection can also occur. Good peri-operative lavages of the donor lungs and the recipient's pleural cavity is important to reduce the presence of infected material. It is often difficult for antibiotics to penetrate the pleural cavity so although infections at a wound site are unusual, once present, they can be difficult to manage and treat. Again, PwCF are at higher risk of infections at anastomotic and surgical sites by the nature of the underlying disease. The antibiotics selected peri-operatively and post-operatively are guided by the patient's response to antibiotic combinations pre-operatively, as well as microbiological sensitivities. Just like other intensive-care patients, post-transplant patients are at high risk of ventilator-associated pneumonia (VAP), and so unless there are contraindications, it is important to work towards extubating the patient as expediently as possible.

CMV (cytomegalovirus) disease used to be a significant concern post-transplant, but the routine use of prophylactic and treatment valgangiclovir combined with surveillance management has significantly reduced the risk of infection or reactivation [86]. A recent study looking at the incidence of CMV infection in heart transplant recipients has estimated the rate of early-onset (<100 days post-transplant) CMV disease at only 2%, compared with late-onset (>100 days post-transplant) at 7.5%, and this is largely thought to be due to the introduction of valganciclovir [87]. EBV (Epstein–Barr virus) mismatches where the donor is positive and the recipient negative, are rare as >95% of the population seroconvert by the time they are 20 years of age. Most recipients undergo a B-cell proliferation 1–3 months post-transplant, but occasionally this can proceed to a post-transplant lymphoproliferative disease (PTLD). Monitoring of EBV levels is generally used as a marker of over-immunosuppression rather than a way of looking for malignant disease. Similarly, with the widespread use of co-trimoxazole as first-line prophylaxis, PCP (pneumocystis pneumonia) – also known as PJP (*pneumocystis jiroveci pneumonia*) – is an unusual finding, with rates in solid organ transplant recipients reduced from 5 to 15% to 0.3–2.6% [88]. Other respiratory viruses that can have significant impact to a transplant recipient includes respiratory syncytial virus (RSV), metapneumovirus, influenza/parainfluenza, adenoviruses and rhinovirus. Any of these can cause a viral pneumonitis, which can in turn inflict permanent damage to the transplanted lungs, either through the inflammatory process of an infection, or by triggering acute rejection or chronic allograft dysfunction (CLAD) [89]. Most of these infections have no direct treatment, and so management remains supportive with the addition of IV methylprednisolone and/or IV immunoglobulin (IVIG) in an effort to prevent rejection which can be triggered by these viral infections [89].

Many PwCF are often sensitised to *Aspergillus fumigatus* and will often be on longterm oral antifungals that will need to continue following transplantation. For all causes, invasive aspergillosis is the most common cause of all invasive fungal infections in lung transplant recipients [90], but it can also be asymptomatic. Often however, it will lead to a more pathogenic process, including causing anastomotic dehiscence and lung function decline without obvious radiographic changes [91]. This process is still not fully understood, which often results in trials of treatment to find the most effective. *A. fumigatus* accounts for 44% of fungal infections in the post-lung transplant population, but other common fungal infections post-transplant include *Candida* (23%), *Scedosporium* (20%), *Mucorales* (3%) and *Cryptococcus* (2%) [92]. Throughout a recipient's lifetime, it is often difficult to tell the difference between rejection and infection as no reliable markers exist. Recipients are subjected to frequent invasive investigations (usually bronchoscopy) especially in the early post-transplant period, requiring washings and biopsies to differentiate. Patients are encouraged to attend their transplant centres as their local referring centre which usually treat patients as having infections rather than consider or have the means to investigate for a diagnosis of rejection. This is especially true for PwCF as they are likely to remain positive for their primary pre-transplant pathogenic bacteria. It is important to keep in mind that they are also susceptible to the same atypical infections as all other lung transplant recipients are, and that even if a diagnosis of infection is correct, it may not be caused by the same causative organisms as per prior to transplantation.

Part of keeping transplant recipients well includes maintaining appropriate prophylactic antibiotic cover. In CF recipients, this often means continuing the oral anti-fungals or nebulised antibiotics they were on pre-transplant for a number of months at least. If these recipients remains well with no positive microbiology, an informed decision to reduce the prophylaxis burden could be considered. All recipients are advised to maintain annual vaccines such as the flu vaccine, but other vaccines should be discussed with transplant centres as not all vaccines are appropriate in the immunosuppressed population.

4.3 Rejection

The first 2 months post-transplant are high risk for acute rejection, as recipient lymphocytes encounter donor antibodies for the first time. However, the risk of death is low with acute cellular rejection (ACR), and this decreases even further with time [93]. Longer term, the risk is of bronchiolitis obliterans syndrome (for which ACR is a risk factor) and CLAD. Unlike most other solid organt transplants (SOT), lung transplantation has always required a fine balance between adequate immunosuppression and the risk of infection. Many patients end up with varying individualised immunosuppression based on the number of rejection episodes against the rate of infections each person has 28% of surviving lung transplant recipients between 2004 and 2015 required treatment for acute rejection in the first year post-discharge [3]. Most recipients will require treatment for acute rejection in the first year post-transplant, usually in the first 6 months [94]. Treatment is usually a short course of high dose IV methylprednisolone (IVMP) for 3–5 days, followed by a tapering course over 2–3 weeks. If a patient suffers from recurrent bouts of acute rejection and treatment adherence is confirmed, then immunosuppression may need to be increased if tolerated renally. Where acute cellular rejection is refractory to standard treatment, other modalities of treatment are available. RATG has variable success but is still used. Total lymphoid irradiation (TLI) and extracorporeal photophoresis are both used with a degree of success in slowing the rate of lung function decline, sometimes halting it altogether [95, 96].

Chronic lung allograft dysfunction (CLAD) remains a major barrier to long-term survival post lung transplantation. Until recently, CLAD and bronchiolitis obliterans syndrome (BOS) were used interchangeably. However, the heterogeneity of the clinical course of CLAD along with highly variable responses to treatment has caused clinicians to review radiology and histology and suggest two distinct phenotypes: BOS and restrictive allograft syndrome (RAS) (also known as restrictive CLAD (rCLAD)). BOS is characterised by an obstructive picture on pulmonary function tests, air trapping on CT imaging, and obliterative bronchiolitis (OB) on histology [97]. RAS is characterised by restrictive results on pulmonary function tests, pleuro-parenchymal infiltrates on CT and fibro-elastosis on biopsies [98]. It is important to differentiate between the two as patients with RAS have an average expected life expectancy of 6–18 months following diagnosis, compared to 3–5 years after diagnosis of BOS [97].

4.4 Malignancy

With improved survival post-transplant, long term complications are increasingly common. Lung transplantation requires higher amounts of immunosuppression compared with most other solid organ transplants, which increases the risk of developing cancer due to impaired anti-tumour immune surveillance and anti-viral activity. Malignancies occur in 18% of patients reaching 5 years of survival, and 28.7% of patients reaching 10 years of survival [99]. Malignancies transmitted from the donor are rare due to the surveillance undertaken at the time of donation [100].

PTLD is diagnosed when EBV levels start to rise in association with an abnormal white cell count, and is more common in lung transplant recipients than most other SOT recipients. It occurs in 2–9% of lung transplant recipients [101, 102]. Early cases (within 1 year of transplantation) typically involve the lungs and occur in recipients who have not previously been exposed to the virus, whereas cases presenting more than 1 year post-transplantation are more likely to involve the gastrointestinal (GI) tract [101]. Radiologically, lymphadenopathy and pulmonary nodules in the peripheral and basal zones are seen on CT [103]. Post-transplant immunosuppression impairs T-cell-specific immunity against EBV but EBV-negative PTLD has also been recognised. Early-onset PTLD is more likely to respond to a reduction in immunosuppression than late-onset as the pathogenesis of the latter is less well understood, but this in turn increases the risk of rejection and graft failure [104]. As a result, prognosis with late-onset PTLD is worse [102, 105]. If reduction in treatment is not the solution, the next option would be rituximab, which induces cell death of B-cells via CD20 which is on the surface of these cells.

Non-melanoma skin cancers are the most common skin cancer for SOT recipients and this is also true in LTx [106, 107]. All lung transplant recipients are advised to monitor their skin for any suspicious changes, and regular review by their GP or a dermatologist is often recommended. They are also cautioned about time spent in the sun and advised to use high factor sun cream liberally. Squamous cell carcinomas (SCCs) are 100–200 times more likely to occur post-lung transplant compared to the general population [107], and they are usually more aggressive with high rates of recurrence [102]. All other forms of skin cancer are more common than the general population but not to the same extent. The increased risk of non-melanoma cancer in all SOT recipients is primarily due to immunosuppression which affects the usual cellular pathways that prevent cancerous growths. With LTx recipients receiving the highest levels of immunosuppression, it is unsurprising that this group of patients have the highest rates of skin cancer. There is also increasing evidence that voriconazole increases the risk of SCC [108] and so it is advised to reduce the length of treatment time if possible and otherwise switch to an alternative anti-fungal that appears to have less of an association with cancer.

Treatment is identical to all other skin cancer treatments, aiming for local excision with complete clearance, but if possible, rates of immunosuppression should be reduced to reduce the risk of recurrence or further skin cancers. Radiotherapy is an alternative option for those who are high risk for surgery or whose cancers have progressed to being inoperable [109]. Monoclonal antibodies have had increasing success in the general population, however, these have not been tried to a great extent in post-transplant recipients due to concerns over their interaction with immunosuppression and risk of graft rejection.

Lung transplant recipients appear to have up to a 5-fold increased risk of lung cancer compared to the general population [110], but the risk is primarily related to pre-transplant risk factors and so there is a higher incidence in those transplanted for COPD or ILD. For PwCF, the risk of developing lung cancer is generally donor-related risk factors or due to immunosuppression as described earlier. When lung cancer does develop, treatment remains challenging as no treatment has been well-studied alongside immunosuppression, and outcomes are often poor.

Although all SOT recipients are at increased risk of developing colorectal cancer, LTx recipients who have CF have a significantly higher incidence, even within the transplant population [111]. This is presumed to be due to the inherent risk of GI malignancy in all PwCF compounded with the increased incidence due to immunosuppression. The US-based CF Foundation have recently published Consensus guidelines for colorectal cancer screening in PwCF which should be followed post-transplant also [112]. Further information on colorectal cancer in CF can be found in the chapter entitled "Digestive System".

5. Conclusions

Although lung transplantation in PwCF has achieved results once thought impossible, there remains substantial opportunity for progress. Avenues for these opportunities include better donor management and organ preservation, improved donor allocation systems to offer organs to those most in need who will also benefit most, optimization of recipients in terms of physiology, GERD management and CFRDM, and prevention of PGD, rejection, and infections. Preoperative pleurodesis and lung resections are not contraindications to lung transplantation, however, strategic planning with CT imaging and availability of experienced team members may reduce complications. While preoperative mechanical ventilation is potentially detrimental, patients should be bridged to lung transplantation with ECMO support, aiming to wake them as soon as is feasible. Bilateral thoracotomy approach is superior to the conventional clamshell cosmetically as well as in regards to wound complications. Elective use of mechanical circulatory support in LTx for CF is now limited to severe secondary pulmonary hypertension or additional cardiac surgery, and in the case of hemodynamic instability or inadequate gas exchange on single lung ventilation, the operation should be performed under ECMO support.

Author details

Prashant N. Mohite*, Kavita Dave, Anna Reed and André R. Simon
Royal Brompton and Harefield NHS Foundation Trust, United Kingdom

*Address all correspondence to: p.mohite@rbht.nhs.uk

References

[1] Yacoub MH, Banner NR, Khaghani A, et al. Heart-lung transplantation for CF and subsequent domino heart transplantation. J Heart Transplant. 1990;9(5):459-467.

[2] Chambers DC, Cherikh WS, Harhay MO, et al. The International Thoracic Organ Transplant Registry of the International Society for Heart and Lung Transplantation. Thirty-sixth adult lung and heart-lung transplantation Report-2019; Focus theme: Donor and recipient size match. J Heart Lung Transplant. 2019;38(10):1042-1055.

[3] Yusen RD, Edwards LB, Kucheryavaya AY, et al. The registry of the International Society for Heart and Lung Transplantation: thirty-first adult lung and heart-lung transplant report--2014; focus theme: retransplantation. J Heart Lung Transplant. 2014;33(10):1009-1024.

[4] Alton EWFW, Armstrong DK, Ashby D, et al. Repeated nebulisation of non-viral CFTR gene therapy in patients with cystic fibrosis: a randomised, double-blind, placebo-controlled, phase 2b trial [published correction appears in Lancet Respir Med. 2015 Sep;3(9):e33]. Lancet Respir Med. 2015;3(9):684-691.

[5] Ratjen F, Hug C, Marigowda G, et al. Efficacy and safety of lumacaftor and ivacaftor in patients aged 6-11 years with cystic fibrosis homozygous for F508del-CFTR: a randomised, placebo-controlled phase 3 trial [published correction appears in Lancet Respir Med. 2017 Aug;5(8):e28]. Lancet Respir Med. 2017;5(7):557-567.

[6] Elborn JS, Ramsey BW, Boyle MP, et al. Efficacy and safety of lumacaftor/ivacaftor combination therapy in patients with cystic fibrosis homozygous for Phe508del CFTR by pulmonary function subgroup: a pooled analysis. Lancet Respir Med. 2016;4(8):617-626.

[7] Kerem E, Reisman J, Corey M, Canny GJ, Levison H. Prediction of mortality in patients with cystic fibrosis. N Engl J Med. 1992;326(18):1187-1191.

[8] Mayer-Hamblett N, Rosenfeld M, Emerson J, Goss CH, Aitken ML. Developing cystic fibrosis lung transplant referral criteria using predictors of 2-year mortality. Am J Respir Crit Care Med. 2002;166(12 Pt 1):1550-1555.

[9] Keogh RH, Seaman SR, Barrett JK, Taylor-Robinson D, Szczesniak R. Dynamic Prediction of Survival in Cystic Fibrosis: A Landmarking Analysis Using UK Patient Registry Data. Epidemiology. 2019;30(1):29-37.

[10] Desai S, Wong H, Sykes J, Stephenson AL, Singer J, Quon BS. Clinical Characteristics and Predictors of Reduced Survival for Adult-diagnosed Cystic Fibrosis. Analysis of the Canadian CF Registry. Ann Am Thorac Soc. 2018;15(10):1177-1185.

[11] Koutsokera A, Varughese RA, Sykes J, et al. Pre-transplant factors associated with mortality after lung transplantation in cystic fibrosis: A systematic review and meta-analysis. J Cyst Fibros. 2019;18(3):407-415.

[12] Weill D, Benden C, Corris PA, et al. A consensus document for the selection of lung transplant candidates: 2014--an update from the Pulmonary Transplantation Council of the International Society for Heart and Lung Transplantation. J Heart Lung Transplant. 2015;34(1):1-15.

[13] Orens JB, Estenne M, Arcasoy S, et al. International guidelines for the selection of lung transplant candidates:

2006 update--a consensus report from the Pulmonary Scientific Council of the International Society for Heart and Lung Transplantation. J Heart Lung Transplant. 2006;25(7):745-755.

[14] Glanville AR, Estenne M. Indications, patient selection and timing of referral for lung transplantation. Eur Respir J. 2003;22(5):845-852.

[15] Hirche TO, Knoop C, Hebestreit H, et al. Practical guidelines: lung transplantation in patients with cystic fibrosis [published correction appears in Pulm Med. 2015;2015:698460]. Pulm Med. 2014;2014:621342.

[16] Kourliouros A, Hogg R, Mehew J, et al. Patient outcomes from time of listing for lung transplantation in the UK: are there disease-specific differences?. Thorax. 2019;74(1):60-68.

[17] Egan TM, Edwards LB. Effect of the lung allocation score on lung transplantation in the United States. J Heart Lung Transplant. 2016;35(4):433-439.

[18] Chen H, Shiboski SC, Golden JA, et al. Impact of the lung allocation score on lung transplantation for pulmonary arterial hypertension. Am J Respir Crit Care Med. 2009;180(5):468-474.

[19] Gottlieb J, Smits J, Schramm R, et al. Lung Transplantation in Germany Since the Introduction of the Lung Allocation Score. Dtsch Arztebl Int. 2017;114(11):179-185.

[20] Merlo CA, Weiss ES, Orens JB, et al. Impact of U.S. Lung Allocation Score on survival after lung transplantation. J Heart Lung Transplant. 2009;28(8):769-775..

[21] Tsuang WM, Vock DM, Copeland CAF, Lederer DJ, Palmer SM. An acute change in lung allocation score and survival after lung transplantation: a cohort study. Ann Intern Med. 2013;158(9):650-657.

[22] Valapour M, Skeans MA, Smith JM, et al. OPTN/SRTR 2015 Annual Data Report: Lung. Am J Transplant. 2017;17 Suppl 1:357-424.

[23] Cardiothoracic Advisory Group (CTAG) on behalf of NHSBT, 2017. Donor lung distribution and allocation. http://odt.nhs.uk/pdf/lung_allocation_policy.pdf (accessed 15 Jun 2020).

[24] https://statistics.eurotransplant.org accessed on 18/06/2020

[25] Van Raemdonck D, Keshavjee S, Levvey B, et al. Donation after circulatory death in lung transplantation-five-year follow-up from ISHLT Registry. J Heart Lung Transplant. 2019;38(12):1235-1245.

[26] Krutsinger D, Reed RM, Blevins A, et al. Lung transplantation from donation after cardiocirculatory death: a systematic review and meta-analysis. J Heart Lung Transplant. 2015;34(5):675-684.

[27] Zhou J, Chen B, Liao H, et al. The Comparable Efficacy of Lung Donation After Circulatory Death and Brain Death: A Systematic Review and Meta-analysis. Transplantation. 2019;103(12):2624-2633.

[28] Miñambres E, Coll E, Duerto J, et al. Effect of an intensive lung donor-management protocol on lung transplantation outcomes. J Heart Lung Transplant. 2014;33:178-184.

[29] Mascia L, Pasero D, Slutsky AS, et al. Effect of a lung protective strategy for organ donors on eligibility and availability of lungs for transplantation: a randomized controlled trial. JAMA. 2010;304:2620-2627.

[30] Mulligan MJ, Sanchez PG, Evans CF, et al. The use of extended criteria donors decreases one-year survival in

high-risk lung recipients: A review of the United Network of Organ Sharing Database. J Thorac Cardiovasc Surg. 2016;152(3):891-898.e2.

[31] Moreno P, Alvarez A, Santos F, et al. Extended recipients but not extended donors are associated with poor outcomes following lung transplantation. Eur J Cardiothorac Surg. 2014;45(6):1040-1047.

[32] Smits JM, van der Bij W, Van Raemdonck D, et al. Defining an extended criteria donor lung: an empirical approach based on the Eurotransplant experience. Transpl Int. 2011;24(4):393-400.

[33] Tian D, Wang Y, Shiiya H, et al. Outcomes of marginal donors for lung transplantation after ex vivo lung perfusion: A systematic review and meta-analysis [published online ahead of print, 2019 Aug 25]. J Thorac Cardiovasc Surg. 2019;S0022-5223(19)31641-1.

[34] Luo Q, Zhu L, Wang Y, Wang L, Lv W, Hu J. The Conversional Efficacy of Ex Vivo Lung Perfusion and Clinical Outcomes in Patients Undergoing Transplantation of Donor Lungs by Ex Vivo Lung Perfusion: A Meta-Analysis. Ann Transplant. 2019;24:647-660.

[35] Chakos A, Ferret P, Muston B, Yan TD, Tian DH. Ex-vivo lung perfusion versus standard protocol lung transplantation-mid-term survival and meta-analysis. Ann Cardiothorac Surg. 2020;9(1):1-9.

[36] Annual Report 2018. http://www.eurotransplant.org

[37] Smits JM, Gottlieb J, Verschuuren E, et al. Impact of donor lung quality on post-transplant recipient outcome in the Lung Allocation Score era in Eurotransplant - a historical prospective study. Transpl Int. 2020;33(5):544-554.

[38] Flume PA, Strange C, Ye X, Ebeling M, Hulsey T, Clark LL. Pneumothorax in cystic fibrosis. Chest. 2005;128(2):720-728.

[39] Flume PA, Mogayzel PJ Jr, Robinson KA, et al. Cystic fibrosis pulmonary guidelines: pulmonary complications: hemoptysis and pneumothorax. Am J Respir Crit Care Med. 2010;182(3):298-306.

[40] Curtis HJ, Bourke SJ, Dark JH, Corris PA. Lung transplantation outcome in cystic fibrosis patients with previous pneumothorax. J Heart Lung Transplant 2005; 24: 865-869.

[41] Belle-van Meerkerk G, de Jong PA, de Valk HW, et al. Pretransplant HRCT Characteristics Are Associated with Worse Outcome of Lung Transplantation for Cystic Fibrosis Patients. PLoS One. 2015;10(12):e0145597.

[42] Shigemura N, Bhama J, Gries CJ, et al. Lung transplantation in patients with prior cardiothoracic surgical procedures. Am J Transplant. 2012;12(5):1249-1255.

[43] Bremner RM, Woo MS, Arroyo H, et al. The effect of pleural adhesions on pediatric cystic fibrosis patients undergoing lung transplantation. Am Surg. 2001;67(12):1136-1139.

[44] Omara M, Okamoto T, Arafat A, Thuita L, Blackstone EH, McCurry KR. Lung transplantation in patients who have undergone prior cardiothoracic procedures. J Heart Lung Transplant. 2016;35(12):1462-1470.

[45] Loeve M, Hop WC, de Bruijne M, et al. Chest computed tomography scores are predictive of survival in patients with cystic fibrosis awaiting lung transplantation. Am J Respir Crit Care Med. 2012;185(10):1096-1103.

[46] Sheikh SI, McCoy KS, Ryan-Wenger NA, Patel A,

Kirkby S. Lobectomy in patients with cystic fibrosis. Can Respir J. 2014;21(4):e63-e66.

[47] Villac Adde F, Vidal Campos S, de Oliveira Braga Teixeira RH, Rodrigues JC. Indications for lung resection surgery and lung transplant in South American children with cystic fibrosis. Paediatr Respir Rev. 2018;25:37-42.

[48] Banga A, Mohanka M, Mullins J, et al. Incidence and variables associated with 30-day mortality after lung transplantation. Clin Transplant. 2019;33(2):e13468.

[49] Banga A, Mohanka M, Mullins J, et al. Hospital length of stay after lung transplantation: Independent predictors and association with early and late survival. J Heart Lung Transplant. 2017;36(3):289-296.

[50] Hayes D Jr, Kopp BT, Preston TJ, et al. Survival of patients with cystic fibrosis on ECMO: analysis of the Extracorporeal Life Support Organization Registry. Int J Clin Exp Med. 2014;7(5):1370-1372.

[51] Fuehner T, Kuehn C, Hadem J, et al. Extracorporeal membrane oxygenation in awake patients as bridge to lung transplantation. Am J Respir Crit Care Med. 2012;185(7):763-768.

[52] Mohite PN, Sabashnikov A, Reed A, et al. Extracorporeal Life Support in "Awake" Patients as a Bridge to Lung Transplant. Thorac Cardiovasc Surg. 2015;63(8):699-705.

[53] de Leval MR, Smyth R, Whitehead B, et al. Heart and lung transplantation for terminal cystic fibrosis. A 4 1/2-year experience. J Thorac Cardiovasc Surg. 1991;101(4):633-642.

[54] Forty J, Hasan A, Gould FK, Corris PA, Dark JH. Single lung transplantation with simultaneous contralateral pneumonectomy for cystic fibrosis. J Heart Lung Transplant. 1994;13(4):727-730

[55] Piotrowski JA, Splittgerber FH, Donovan TJ, Ratjen F, Zerkowski HR. Single-lung transplantation in a patient with cystic fibrosis and an asymmetric thorax. Ann Thorac Surg. 1997;64(5): 1456-1459.

[56] Mitilian D, Sage E, Puyo P, et al. Techniques and results of lobar lung transplantations. Eur J Cardiothorac Surg. 2014;45(2):365-370.

[57] Marasco SF, Than S, Keating D, et al. Cadaveric lobar lung transplantation: technical aspects. Ann Thorac Surg. 2012;93(6):1836-1842.

[58] Couetil JP, Tolan MJ, Loulmet DF, et al. Pulmonary bipartitioning and lobar transplantation: a new approach to donor organ shortage. J Thorac Cardiovasc Surg. 1997;113(3):529-537.

[59] Barbers RG. Cystic fibrosis: bilateral living lobar versus cadaveric lung transplantation. Am J Med Sci. 1998;315(3):155-160.

[60] Starnes VA, Bowdish ME, Woo MS, et al. A decade of living lobar lung transplantation: recipient outcomes. J Thorac Cardiovasc Surg. 2004;127(1):114-122.

[61] Marczin N, Popov AF, Zych B, et al. Outcomes of minimally invasive lung transplantation in a single centre: the routine approach for the future or do we still need clamshell incision?. Interact Cardiovasc Thorac Surg. 2016;22(5):537-545.

[62] Pochettino A, Augoustides JG, Kowalchuk DA, Watcha SM, Cowie D, Jobes DR. Cardiopulmonary bypass for lung transplantation in cystic fibrosis: pilot evaluation of perioperative outcome. J Cardiothorac Vasc Anesth. 2007;21(2):208-211.

[63] Liu Y, Liu Y, Su L, Jiang SJ. Recipient-related clinical risk factors for primary graft dysfunction after lung transplantation: a systematic review and meta-analysis. PLoS One. 2014;9(3):e92773.

[64] Jauregui A, Deu M, Romero L, et al. Lung Transplantation in Cystic Fibrosis and the Impact of Extracorporeal Circulation. El trasplante pulmonar en la fibrosis quística y la influencia de la circulación extracorpórca. Arch Bronconeumol. 2018;54(6):313-319.

[65] Aeba R, Griffith BP, Kormos RL, et al. Effect of cardiopulmonary bypass on early graft dysfunction in clinical lung transplantation. Ann Thorac Surg. 1994;57(3):715-722.

[66] Gammie JS, Cheul Lee J, Pham SM, et al. Cardiopulmonary bypass is associated with early allograft dysfunction but not death after double-lung transplantation. J Thorac Cardiovasc Surg. 1998;115(5):990-997.

[67] Mohite PN, Sabashnikov A, Patil NP, et al. The role of cardiopulmonary bypass in lung transplantation. Clin Transplant. 2016;30(3):202-209.

[68] Magouliotis DE, Tasiopoulou VS, Svokos AA, Svokos KA, Zacharoulis D. Extracorporeal membrane oxygenation versus cardiopulmonary bypass during lung transplantation: a meta-analysis. Gen Thorac Cardiovasc Surg. 2018;66(1):38-47.

[69] Gottlieb J, Mattner F, Weissbrodt H, et al. Impact of graft colonization with gram-negative bacteria after lung transplantation on the development of bronchiolitis obliterans syndrome in recipients with cystic fibrosis. Respir Med. 2009;103(5):743-749.

[70] Calabrese F, Lunardi F, Nannini N, et al. Higher Risk of Acute Cellular Rejection in Lung Transplant Recipients with Cystic Fibrosis. Ann Transplant. 2015;20:769-776.

[71] Lobo LJ, Aris RM, Schmitz J, Neuringer IP. Donor-specific antibodies are associated with antibody-mediated rejection, acute cellular rejection, bronchiolitis obliterans syndrome, and cystic fibrosis after lung transplantation. J Heart Lung Transplant. 2013;32(1):70-77.

[72] Novick RJ, Stitt LW, Al-Kattan K, et al. Pulmonary retransplantation: predictors of graft function and survival in 230 patients. Pulmonary Retransplant Registry. Ann Thorac Surg. 1998;65(1):227-234.

[73] Aigner C, Jaksch P, Taghavi S, et al. Pulmonary retransplantation: is it worth the effort? A long-term analysis of 46 cases. J Heart Lung Transplant. 2008;27(1):60-65.

[74] Thomas M, Belli EV, Rawal B, Agnew RC, Landolfo KP. Survival After Lung Retransplantation in the United States in the Current Era (2004 to 2013): Better or Worse?. Ann Thorac Surg. 2015;100(2):452-457.

[75] Strueber M, Fischer S, Gottlieb J, et al. Long-term outcome after pulmonary retransplantation. J Thorac Cardiovasc Surg. 2006;132(2):407-412.

[76] Chambers DC, Cherikh WS, Harhay MO, Hayes D, Hsich E, Khush KK, Meiser B, Potena L, Rossano JW, Toll AE, et al. The International Thoracic Organ Transplant Registry of the International Society for Heart and Lung Transplantation: Thirty-sixth adult lung and heart–lung transplantation Report—2019; Focus theme: Donor and recipient size match. J Hear Lung Transplant 2019;38(10):1042-1055.

[77] Yusen RD, Edwards LB, Kucheryavaya AY, Benden C,

Dipchand AI, Dobbels F, Goldfarb SB, Levvey BJ, Lund LH, Meiser B, et al. The Registry of the International Society for Heart and Lung Transplantation: Thirty-first Adult Lung and Heart–Lung Transplant Report—2014; Focus Theme: Retransplantation. J Hear Lung Transplant 2014;33(10):1009-1024.

[78] Yusen RD, Edwards LB, Dipchand AI, Goldfarb SB, Kucheryavaya AY, Levvey BJ, Lund LH, Meiser B, Rossano JW, Stehlik J. The Registry of the International Society for Heart and Lung Transplantation: Thirty-third Adult Lung and Heart–Lung Transplant Report—2016; Focus Theme: Primary Diagnostic Indications for Transplant. J Hear Lung Transplant 2016;35(10):1170-1184.

[79] Christie JD, Kotloff RM, Pochettino A, Arcasoy SM, Rosengard BR, Landis JR, Kimmel SE. Clinical Risk Factors for Primary Graft Failure Following Lung Transplantation. Chest 2003;124(4):1232-1241.

[80] Whitson BA, Nath DS, Johnson AC, Walker AR, Prekker ME, Radosevich DM, Herrington CS, Dahlberg PS. Risk factors for primary graft dysfunction after lung transplantation. J Thorac Cardiovasc Surg 2006;131(1):73-80.

[81] Whitson BA, Prekker ME, Herrington CS, Whelan TPM, Radosevich DM, Hertz MI, Dahlberg PS. Primary graft dysfunction and long-term pulmonary function after lung transplantation. J Heart Lung Transplant 2007;26(10):1004-1011.

[82] Huang HJ, Yusen RD, Meyers BF, Walter MJ, Mohanakumar T, Patterson GA, Trulock EP, Hachem RR. Late primary graft dysfunction after lung transplantation and bronchiolitis obliterans syndrome. Am J Transplant 2008;8(11):2454-2462.

[83] Gilljam M, Scherstén H, Silverborn M, Jönsson B, Ericsson Hollsing A. Lung transplantation in patients with cystic fibrosis and Mycobacterium abscessus infection. J Cyst Fibros 2010;9(4):272-276.

[84] Raats D, Lorent N, Saegeman V, Vos R, van Ingen J, Verleden G, Van Raemdonck D, Dupont L. Successful lung transplantation for chronic Mycobacterium abscessus infection in advanced cystic fibrosis, a case series. Transpl Infect Dis 2019;21(2):e13046.

[85] Lobo LJ, Chang LC, Esther CR, Gilligan PH, Tulu Z, Noone PG. Lung transplant outcomes in cystic fibrosis patients with pre-operative Mycobacterium abscessus respiratory infections. Clin Transplant 2013;27(4):523-529.

[86] Johansson I, Mårtensson G, Nyström U, Nasic S, Andersson R. Lower incidence of CMV infection and acute rejections with valganciclovir prophylaxis in lung transplant recipients. BMC Infect Dis 2013;13(1):582.

[87] Santos CAQ, Brennan DC, Fraser VJ, Olsen MA. Incidence, Risk Factors, and Outcomes of Delayed-Onset Cytomegalovirus Disease in a Large, Retrospective Cohort of Heart Transplant Recipients. Transplant Proc 2014;46(10):3585-3592.

[88] Iriart X, Bouar M Le, Kamar N, Berry A. Pneumocystis Pneumonia in Solid-Organ Transplant Recipients. J fungi (Basel, Switzerland) 2015;1(3):293-331.

[89] Shah P, McDyer J. Viral Infections in Lung Transplant Recipients. Semin Respir Crit Care Med 2010;31(02):243-254.

[90] Pappas PG, Alexander BD, Andes DR, Hadley S, Kauffman CA, Freifeld A, Anaissie EJ, Brumble LM, Herwaldt L, Ito J, et al. Invasive Fungal Infections among Organ Transplant

Recipients: Results of the Transplant-Associated Infection Surveillance Network (TRANSNET). Clin Infect Dis 2010;50(8):1101-1111.

[91] Kosmidis C, Denning DW. The clinical spectrum of pulmonary aspergillosis. Thorax 2015;70(3):270-277.

[92] Kennedy CC, Razonable RR. Fungal Infections After Lung Transplantation. Clin Chest Med 2017;38(3):511-520.

[93] Benzimra M, Calligaro GL, Glanville AR. Acute rejection. J Thorac Dis 2017;9(12):5440-5457.

[94] Burton CM, Iversen M, Scheike T, Carlsen J, Andersen CB. Minimal acute cellular rejection remains prevalent up to 2 years after lung transplantation: a retrospective analysis of 2697 transbronchial biopsies. Transplantation 2008;85(4):547-553.

[95] Miller R, Hartog B, Frew J, Parry G, Fisher A, Corris P, Meachery G, Lordan J. Total Lymphoid Irradiation (TLI) for the Management of Bronchiolitis Obliterans Syndrome (BOS) Post Lung Transplant: A Single Centre Experience. J Hear Lung Transplant 2016;35(4):S70.

[96] Isenring B, Robinson C, Buergi U, Schuurmans MM, Kohler M, Huber LC, Benden C. Lung transplant recipients on long-term extracorporeal photopheresis. Clin Transplant 2017;31(10).

[97] Verleden SE, Vos R, Vanaudenaerde BM, Verleden GM. Chronic lung allograft dysfunction phenotypes and treatment. J Thorac Dis 2017;9(8):2650-2659.

[98] Sato M, Waddell TK, Wagnetz U, Roberts HC, Hwang DM, Haroon A, Wagnetz D, Chaparro C, Singer LG, Hutcheon MA, et al. Restrictive allograft syndrome (RAS): A novel form of chronic lung allograft dysfunction. J Hear Lung Transplant 2011;30(7):735-742.

[99] Yusen RD, Edwards LB, Kucheryavaya AY, Benden C, Dipchand AI, Goldfarb SB, Levvey BJ, Lund LH, Meiser B, Rossano JW, et al. The Registry of the International Society for Heart and Lung Transplantation: Thirty-second Official Adult Lung and Heart-Lung Transplantation Report--2015; Focus Theme: Early Graft Failure. J Heart Lung Transplant 2015;34(10):1264-1277.

[100] Myron Kauffman H, McBride MA, Cherikh WS, Spain PC, Marks WH, Roza AM. Transplant tumor registry: donor related malignancies. Transplantation 2002;74(3):358-362.

[101] Kremer BE, Reshef R, Misleh JG, Christie JD, Ahya VN, Blumenthal NP, Kotloff RM, Hadjiliadis D, Stadtmauer EA, Schuster SJ, et al. Post-transplant lymphoproliferative disorder after lung transplantation: A review of 35 cases. J Hear Lung Transplant 2012;31(3):296-304.

[102] Shtraichman O, Ahya VN. Malignancy after lung transplantation. Ann Transl Med 2020;8(6):416-416.

[103] Carignan S, Staples CA, Müller NL. Intrathoracic lymphoproliferative disorders in the immunocompromised patient: CT findings. Radiology 1995;197(1):53-58.

[104] Muchtar E, Kramer MR, Vidal L, Ram R, Gurion R, Rosenblat Y, Bakal I, Shpilberg O. Posttransplantation lymphoproliferative disorder in lung transplant recipients: a 15-year single institution experience. Transplantation 2013;96(7):657-663.

[105] Leyssens A, Dierickx D, Verbeken EK, Tousseyn T, Verleden SE, Vanaudenaerde BM, Dupont LJ, Yserbyt J, Verleden GM, Van Raemdonck DE, et al. Post-transplant lymphoproliferative

disease in lung transplantation: A nested case-control study. Clin Transplant 2017;31(7):e12983.

[106] Berastegui C, LaPorta R, López-Meseguer M, Romero L, Gómez-Ollés S, Riera J, Monforte V, Sáez B, Bravo C, Roman A, et al. Epidemiology and Risk Factors for Cancer After Lung Transplantation. Transplant Proc 2017;49(10):2285-2291.

[107] Rashtak S, Dierkhising RA, Kremers WK, Peters SG, Cassivi SD, Otley CC. Incidence and risk factors for skin cancer following lung transplantation. J Am Acad Dermatol 2015;72(1):92-98.

[108] Hamandi B, Fegbeutel C, Silveira FP, Verschuuren EA, Younus M, Mo J, Yan J, Ussetti P, Chin-Hong P V, Solé A, et al. Voriconazole and squamous cell carcinoma after lung transplantation: A multicenter study. Am J Transplant 2018;18(1):113-124.

[109] O'Reilly Zwald F, Brown M. Skin cancer in solid organ transplant recipients: advances in therapy and management: part II. Management of skin cancer in solid organ transplant recipients. J Am Acad Dermatol 2011;65(2):263-279.

[110] Triplette M, Crothers K, Mahale P, Yanik EL, Valapour M, Lynch CF, Schabath MB, Castenson D, Engels EA. Risk of lung cancer in lung transplant recipients in the United States. Am J Transplant 2019;19(5):1478-1490.

[111] Safaeian M, Robbins HA, Berndt SI, Lynch CF, Fraumeni JF, Engels EA. Risk of Colorectal Cancer After Solid Organ Transplantation in the United States. Am J Transplant 2016;16(3):960-967.

[112] Hadjiliadis D, Khoruts A, Zauber AG, Hempstead SE, Maisonneuve P, Lowenfels AB, Cystic Fibrosis Colorectal Cancer Screening Task Force. Cystic Fibrosis Colorectal Cancer Screening Consensus Recommendations. Gastroenterology 2018;154(3):736-745.e14.

Chapter 6

Recent Advances in Targeted Genetic Medicines for Cystic Fibrosis

Salsabil Elboraie, Konstantinos N. Kafetzis, Rajeev Shrivastava and Aristides D. Tagalakis

Abstract

The cystic fibrosis transmembrane conductance regulator (*CFTR*) gene was discovered just over 30 years ago, and soon after, gene therapy for cystic fibrosis (CF) has been rapidly and continually developing. Recently, novel gene therapy strategies have been developed, including mRNA delivery, genome editing, and mRNA repair; all these strategies are collectively named "genetic medicines." The last quarter of the century showed a significant boost in the development of viral and nonviral vectors to deliver genetic treatment. This chapter will provide a brief overview of the *CFTR* gene and its different classes of mutations as well as a review of the different genetic therapeutic options that are under research. Later in this chapter, drugs that target different *CFTR* mutation classes and are currently approved to treat CF patients will be briefly presented.

Keywords: cystic fibrosis, CFTR, gene therapy, CRISPR/Cas9, mRNA therapy, gene editing, gene delivery, viral vectors, nonviral vectors, CF animal models, CF drugs

1. Introduction

CF is an autosomal recessive genetic disorder and is caused by mutations in both copies of *CFTR*. The *CFTR* gene is found on chromosome 7, on the long arm at position q31.2 from bp 116,907,253 to bp 117,095,955. *CFTR* consists of 27 exons, whereas the CFTR protein has 1480 amino acids with a molecular mass of 168,138 Da [1].

The *CFTR* gene encodes a protein that is an ATP-gated chloride and bicarbonate channel. It is located only on the apical membrane of the airway, intestinal, and exocrine glands epithelium. The CFTR protein undergoes different steps of post-translational modifications and trafficking inside the epithelial cells (**Figure 1**). The CFTR protein structure consists of four main domains: an extracellular domain, a transmembrane domain, a nuclear binding domain (NBD), and the regulatory domain (R domain) (**Figure 2**) [2].

1. **Extracellular domain**: It comprises of small loops that connect the transmembrane proteins, e.g., (M1 and M2), (M3 and M4), (M5 and M6), etc.

2. **Transmembrane domain**: It consists of two groups; each of them consists of six membrane-bound regions that are each connected to a nuclear binding

IntechOpen

domain (NBD). It was found that it plays a major role in the pore function of the membrane.

3. **NBD domain (NBD; NBD1 and NBD2)**: It is responsible for ATP binding.

4. **Regulatory domain (R domain)**: It consists of numerous charged amino acids, and it is phosphorylated and activated by protein kinase A.

The CFTR transport mechanism depends on two membrane-spanning domains (MSD) and two nucleotide-binding domains (NBD). The cycle of the transport of the chloride ions starts with the phosphorylation of the R domain that activates the channel. This step will start the ATP ligation to the NBD and the subsequent conformational changes and dimerization. This step will provide the energy for the release of the chloride ions across the cellular membrane. Once ATP is hydrolyzed, the NBD is destabilized, releasing ADP and phosphates; this results in the protein regaining its basal state. This cycle is called the ATP switch model of CFTR [3].

The *CFTR* mutations can be classified into six main classes based on their effect on the synthesis and/or function of the encoded protein. More recently, a Class VII has been added (**Figure 3**) [5, 6].

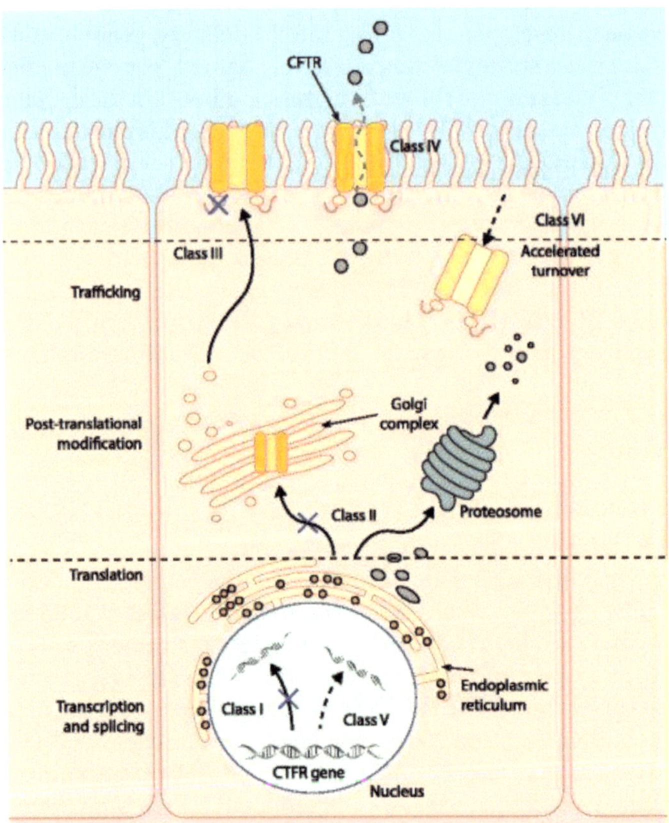

Figure 1.
The physiological process of CFTR *transcription and cellular processing of the protein inside the cells. The process starts with the mRNA transcription in the nucleus, and then the mRNA leaves the nucleus and is translated by ribosomes in the endoplasmic reticulum to protein. Chaperone proteins facilitate folding of the new CFTR proteins. The CFTR protein next undergoes post-translational modifications in the Golgi apparatus such as glycosylation, ubiquitination, SUMOylation, and phosphorylation and is then transported to the epithelial cell surface [4].*

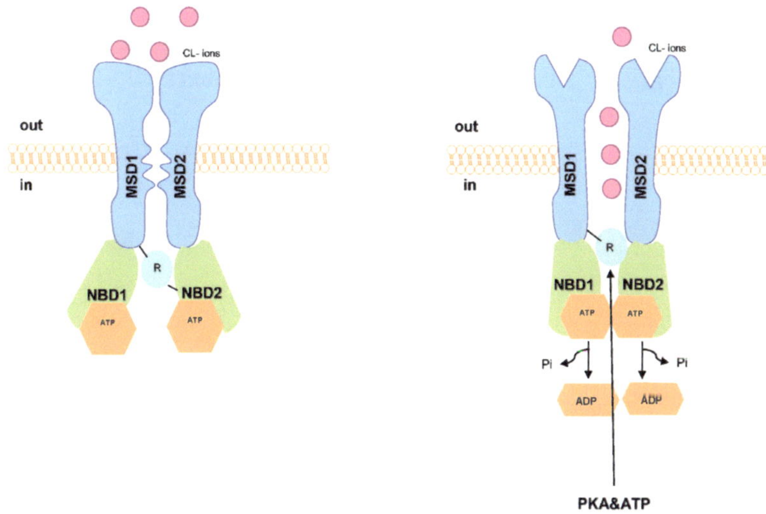

Figure 2.
This figure illustrates the composition of the CFTR chloride channels (at rest and when activated) in the apical epithelial membranes. It is composed of different domains including the MSD, NBD, and the R domains.

Class I mutations result in a partial or complete lack of production of a functional CFTR protein. Those mutations are due to the introduction of a premature termination codon (PTC). This class includes mutations such as p.Gly542X, p.Arg553X, and p.Trp1282X. The p.Gly542X mutation is the most common mutation of this class worldwide.

Class II mutations are associated with abnormal trafficking of the CFTR protein due to misfolding of the protein. These mutations occur in any domain of the CFTR protein and can lead to either a partial reduction (p.Leu206Trp) or complete absence of the mature CFTR protein (p.Arg1066Cys). The F508del (p.Phe508del) is the most common mutation worldwide, and it has been demonstrated that it leads to instability of the NBD1 domain and alters the CFTR assembly.

Class III mutations are missense mutations frequently located in the ATP binding domains (NBD1 and NBD2). They are also known as gating mutations since in this type there is a defective channel gating. There is production of CFTR, which is efficiently transported to the cell membrane at normal levels, but the protein is resistant to activation by protein kinase A and cannot exhibit channel gating function (e.g., p.Gly178Arg and p.Gly551Asp).

Class IV mutations are missense mutations located in the membrane domains, which are responsible for the formation of the channel pores. The protein can still efficiently reach the membrane but with reduced channel conductance (e.g., p.Arg117His and p.Arg334Trp).

Class V mutations reduce the amount of functional CFTR protein. Nonfunctioning proteins are produced due to alternative splicing. Moreover, as a result of amino acid substitution, there is less protein maturation, reducing the amount of functional CFTR that reaches the cell surface. Consequently, the reduced numbers of CFTR channels lead to the subsequent loss of chloride transport (e.g., c.3272-26A>G). Direct RNA analysis is not routinely performed and this in turn leads in underestimation of the number of mutations causing splicing defects.

Class VI mutations result in a protein that is unstable, degrades easily, and has abnormally fast turnover rates due to the truncated C terminus of the protein (e.g., p.Lys684fs and p.Gln1412X).

Finally, **Class VII mutations** are a subtype of Class I mutations with no messenger RNA (mRNA) transcription [7]. The outcome is the same as that of class I mutations, i.e., complete absence of CFTR protein which cannot be treated by the CFTR correctors.

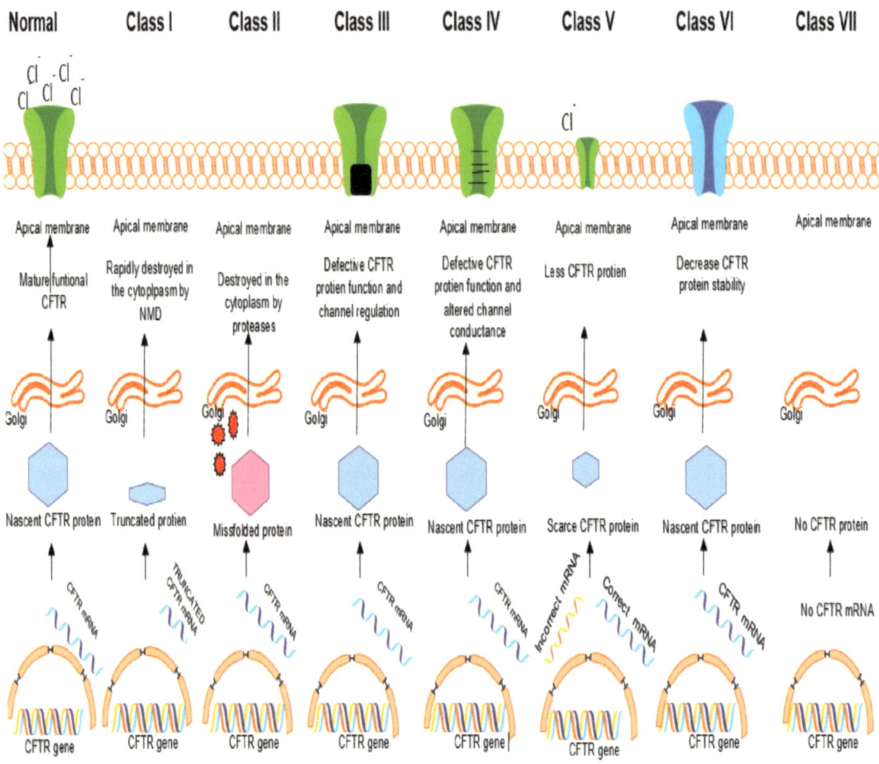

Figure 3.
This figure describes the different classes of CF according to the production of the encoded CFTR protein.

2. Genetic medicine

Although there are some approved drugs for specific patients who harbor certain mutations, genetic medicine is important as it offers the ultimate treatment for all CF mutations and can benefit every CF patient [8]. There are multiple genetic strategies that are currently under investigation for the treatment of CF. They can be summarized as follows (**Figure 4**).

1. **Gene therapy**: Here, the correct copy of the *CFTR* gene is delivered to the diseased CF cells using either viral or nonviral vectors such as nanocomplexes.

2. **Gene editing (repair)**: This technique aims to correct the mutant *CFTR* allele by cutting the double strand DNA and correct the existing mutations inside the cells at the DNA level.

3. **mRNA-based therapeutics**: RNA oligonucleotides are delivered to the cytoplasm and repair the defective CFTR mRNA.

4. **mRNA therapy**: Wild-type CFTR mRNA is delivered to the cytoplasm of the cell, resulting in the production of normal CFTR protein [8].

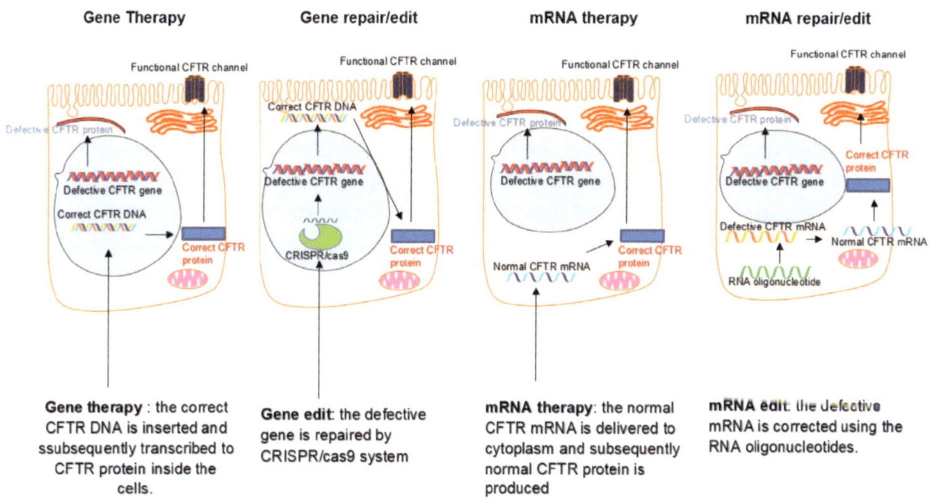

Figure 4.
This figure illustrates the different genetic medicine strategies for gene treatment of the CF mutations. It includes gene therapy, gene editing, mRNA repair, and mRNA therapy.

2.1 Gene therapy

Gene therapy is currently the most advanced and promising field of CF genetic medicine. For a long time, the main obstacle of this approach has been the absence of an efficient delivery system for the lung. The barriers (intracellular or extracellular) that are there to protect us from viruses and bacteria also prevent the uptake of different gene treatments via inhalation. The barriers also include the nuclear membrane which prevents the passage of the genetic materials from the cytoplasm to the nucleus. Other obstacles include airway mucus, mucociliary clearance, CF mucopurulent sputum, and the humoral and cellular immune responses. All these hinder the efficiency and the effectiveness of gene therapy as a treatment for CF [8].

Vectors can be classified broadly into two categories: viral and nonviral [9]. Viral vectors include adenoviruses and adeno-associated viruses (AAV). Both viruses can infect the lung cells efficiently and carry specific proteins in their cell surface to overcome the lung's natural defense systems [10]. However, any preexisting immunity toward the viruses will render them useless. Even if there is no previous immunity, the repeated administration of the virus will eventually lead to the development of immunity toward it and limit its success. However, recent preclinical studies in animals showed that multiple administrations of lentiviral vectors in immunocompetent lungs are effective [10]. Although some adenoviral clinical trials showed partial correction of the chloride transport in CF nasal epithelium by measuring the potential difference between the outer and inner cell membranes, this correction was only recorded after the nasal epithelium was damaged and removed during delivery [10].

Due to the simple structure of the nonviral vectors, they do not usually induce immune reactions inside the body [8]. The UK CF Gene Therapy Consortium (GTC) was formed from three groups in Edinburgh, London, and Oxford. Their aim was to share expertise to assess gene therapy and its ability to stop the progression of CF lung disease. After extensive research, they concluded that the nonviral cationic lipid formulation GL67A combined with the modified pGM169 plasmid (which encodes a CpG-free and codon-optimized CFTR) can produce some improvements in spirometry assessments in animals and even longer duration of response of up to 1 month [8]. In a randomized double-blind phase IIb trial, conducted on 120 patients with different mutations in the UK, it was found that pGM169/GL67A was associated with a small but statistically significant stabilization of lung function in the patients [11]. In addition, the safety of this nonviral system was validated following 12 monthly administrations.

Another promising viral vector that has been investigated is the lentivirus. However, because this virus lacks the lung tropism, it must be combined with another virus in order to transduce the lung cells. The VSV-G protein is commonly used for this purpose, but others like the HA protein from the influenza virus and the F and HN proteins from the Sendai virus (**Figure 5**) have also been used [12].

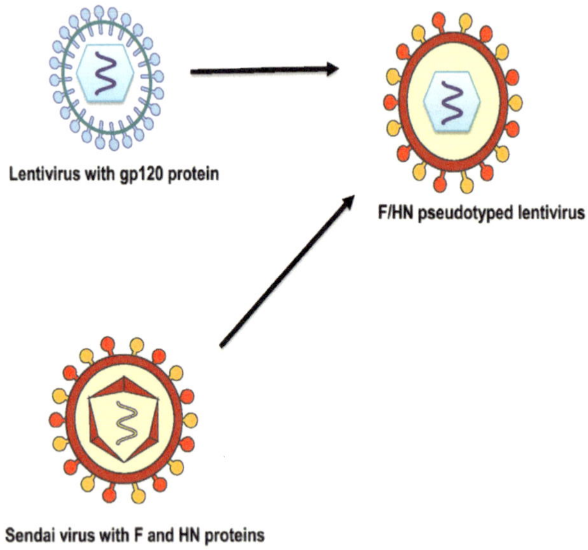

Figure 5.
This figure shows the F/HN pseudotyped lentiviral vector. The virus loses its gp120 protein which originally enables it to enter the T-cells but it gains the HN envelope proteins from the Sendai virus to facilitate its transduction inside the lung epithelial cells.

It has been reported in murines that one dose of lentivirus leads to life-long stable expression of luciferase (almost for 2 years). In addition, repeated administrations of the vector (10 daily doses, or three administrations at monthly intervals) did not cause a significant immune response. In a comparison between the GL67A/pGM169 and the lentivirus, it was found that the lentivirus is a much more effective form of gene therapy [8, 10].

At the end of 2017, the preparation for a clinical trial of a F/HN-pseudotyped lentivirus was announced [8]. This clinical trial will be a single-dose, double-blinded, dose-escalating phase I/IIa safety, and efficacy study. In a preliminary study, for the preparation of this clinical trial, it was predicted that only between 5 and 25% of the lung epithelial cells will need to be corrected in order to provide a clinical level of correction [13].

The human bocavirus virus-1 (HBoV1) is a parvovirus which efficiently infects the human airway epithelium. It was successfully recombined with an adenovirus to give a chimeric rAAV2/HBoV1 virus that was able to deliver a full-length *CFTR* gene coding sequence in CF human epithelial cells [14].

Marked progress in the development of vectors for airway gene delivery, along with a better understanding of CF pathophysiology and the presence of new animal models, has increased the possibility and the hope of gene therapy for CF. However, some obstacles to overcome include the percentage of the lung epithelial cells that need to be corrected to restore physiological function, as well as the limited life span of the ciliated epithelium of the lung. In addition, repeated dosing will require a better understanding of the immune system and the use of immune modulators. Regardless of the strategy, the benefit of a gene therapy approach will ultimately be realized in well-designed CF clinical trials [11].

2.2 Gene editing

Gene editing is an advanced form of genetic engineering which enables the insertion, deletion, or change of the nucleotide sequence of any living organism. It certainly gives the promise of providing therapy for diseases that were previously considered untreatable or difficult to treat. The field of genome-editing technologies is rapidly evolving and progressing, and the newer techniques seem to be more promising [15]. Gene editing was originally developed in the 1980s by Capecchi, Evans, and Smithies (awarded the 2007 Nobel Prize in Physiology or Medicine) but was mainly used in mice and pigs. The outstanding discovery that editing efficiency is increased at the site of double-stranded breaks (DSBs) made it possible to use the technique in larger studies of animal models and human cells. However, a method to create specific breaks at a certain genomic location with minimal off-target effects, insertions, and deletions in the DNA sequence had yet to be discovered [15].

In 2005, the development of fully programmable zinc finger nucleases (ZFNs) and their ability to perform this exact task led to its use in research extensively, but the limitation was the inefficiency and high cost of the ZFNs technology [16]. In 2009, the emergence of TAL-effector nucleases (TALENs) increased the gene editing specificity and the ease of design and production [16]. However, in 2013, the development of the clustered regularly interspaced short palindromic repeats/CRISPR-associated protein 9 (CRISPR/Cas9) system has revolutionized gene editing as a research method that can be used by many groups worldwide [16].

CRISPR is an adaptive immunity function in bacteria like *Streptococcus pyogenes* through which they can defend themselves against the bacteriophage virus' DNA or RNA. The main function of the CRISPR system inside the bacteria is to act as a molecular immunity protective mechanism to keep a copy of previous bacteriophage infections, in the form of a short sequence target of DNA or RNA molecules, inside the cytoplasm of the bacteria, allowing a more rapid identification and elimination of foreign DNA from the cytoplasm [17].

2.2.1 CRISPR/Cas9 system

Generally, the CRISPR/Cas9 system is composed of (**Figure 6**) the following:

1. The cas9 endonuclease that is capable of binding and unwinding the DNA helix and cleave any sequence complimentary to the guide RNA attached to it.

2. The guide RNA molecule (gRNA) that is designed to bind to the desired sequence and direct the Cas9 endonuclease. Usually, it is a short segment about 20 nucleotides long.

3. A template DNA, to achieve the repair of the DSB with homology directed repair (HDR) rather than nonhomologous end joining repair (NHEJ).

The ribonucleoprotein complex of Cas9 and sgRNA first scans the DNA, anneals to the complementary DNA sequence and then makes a double strand cut before the sequence of the protospacer-associated motif (PAM) (it is a part of the DNA sequence ~2–6 base pair long immediately downstream of the sequence targeted by the Cas9 nuclease and it is essential for the Cas9 endonuclease function) [18].

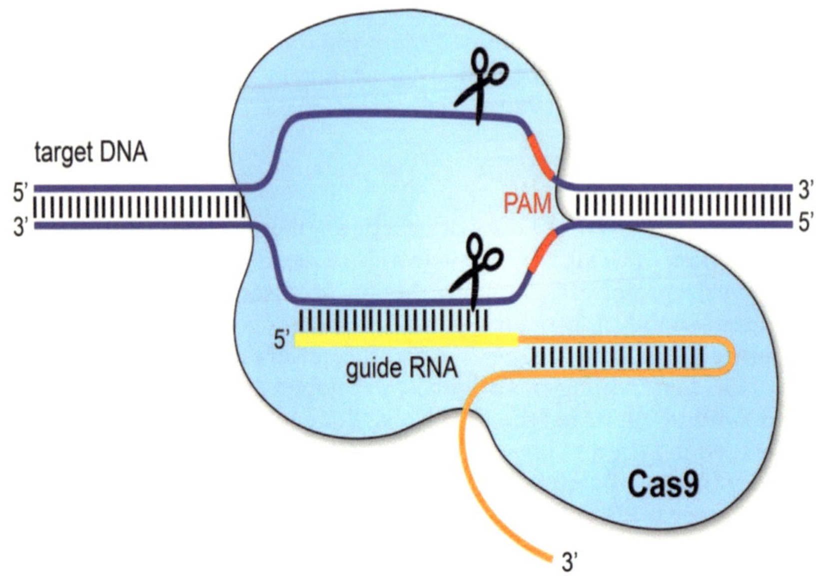

Figure 6.
This figure illustrates the composition of the CRISPR/Cas 9 system [19].

The application of this system for the editing of the genomes is quite simple, efficient, multiplexed, applicable in many species, and relatively affordable compared to other forms of gene editing. In addition, this system can be modified to perform activation or repression of certain genes, and the Cas enzymes can be fused to epigenetic modifiers to create programmable epigenome-engineering tools [20].

A more advanced approach of genome editing is the base editing technique (BE), a newer approach to gene editing that achieves the direct and programmable conversion of one DNA base pair to another DNA base pair chemically, using specific enzymes, without inducing a DSB [21]. It was proposed that different base editors were needed to make more efficient and specific conversion of nucleotides with minimal off-target effects, e.g., the conversion of G: C to A: T by using the third-generation base editor (BE3) [21].

Typically, BE3 contains (**Figure** 7):

1. A catalytically inactive dCas9 that binds only to DNA but is not able to cut the strand. It is only capable of creating a DNA bubble at a guide RNA-specified region.

2. A cytidine deaminase enzyme that changes cytidine to uracil within a 3–5 nucleotide window of the single-stranded DNA bubble, e.g. APOBEC1 (Apolipoprotein B mRNA editing enzyme, catalytic polypeptide-like 1 enzyme).

3. A uracil glycosylase inhibitor (UGI) that inhibits the automatic cellular repair mechanisms by inhibiting the base excision, therefore improving the efficiency of the BE technique.

4. Nickase activity: to make a cut only in one strand of the DNA in order to achieve manipulation of the cellular mismatch repair innate mechanisms of the cells to replace the G-containing DNA strand.

These components combine to achieve a permanent C to T (or G to A) conversion in the cells with minimal or lack of in-del formation [21].

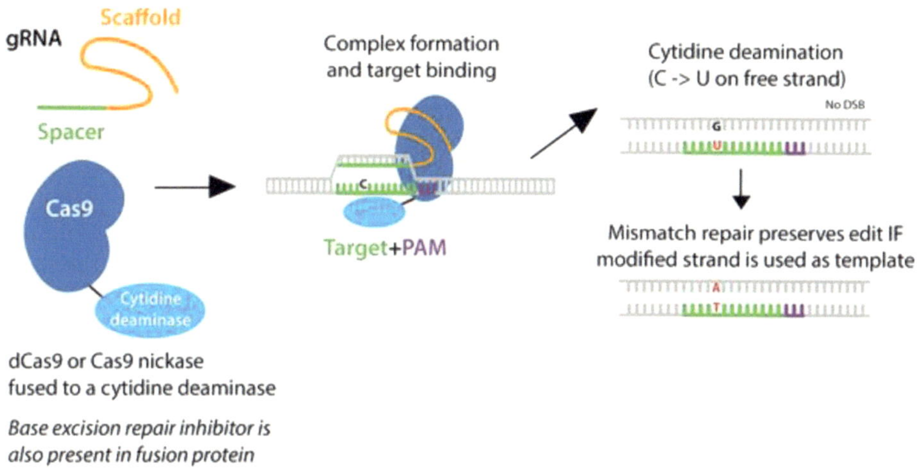

Figure 7.
This figure describes the different components and the mechanism of action of base editing converting G: C to A: T [22].

Moreover, additional modifications have been made to BEs to limit off-target effects (e.g., Hypa-BE3), decrease bystander effects (e.g., YE1-BE3, YE2-BE3), increase the editing window (BE-PLUS), and improve intracellular expression (BE4max) [23].

A recent technique (late 2017) is the use of Adenine base editor (ABE) which is able to convert A: T to G: C by using an adenine deaminase enzyme such as E. coli TAD-A, human ADAR2, mouse ADA, and human ADAT2 [22]. The adenine base is converted to inosine by deamination. Inosine is then treated as guanine by cell polymerases, therefore pairing it with cytidine in the opposite strand and ultimately converting A: T to G: C. The ABE also consists of a guide RNA, a catalytically impaired Cas9 and an adenine deaminase enzyme such as E. coli TAD-A (**Figure 8**).

Therefore, these base editors (both ABEs and BEs) revolutionize the field of genome editing and can position all the transitional DNA bases at specific loci in different cells with a minimum of harmful by-products [24].

In CF, CRISPR/Cas9 was used to correct the F508del mutation, which resulted in recovery of the functions of CFTR in human gastrointestinal tract stem cells in

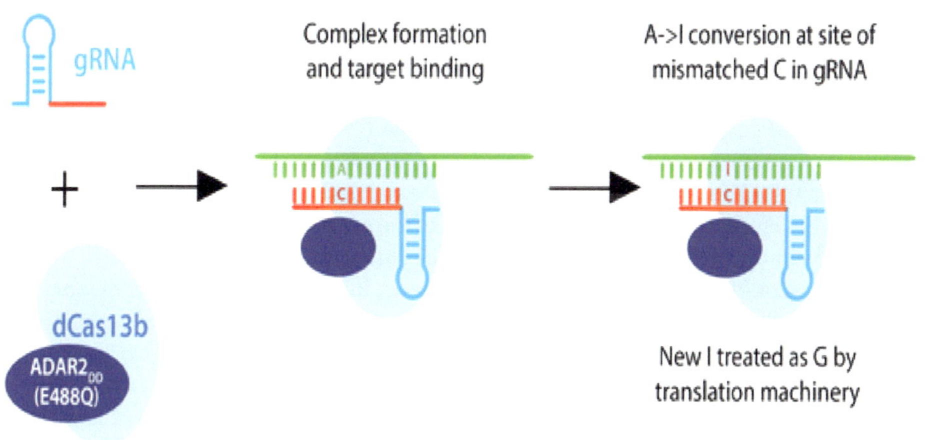

Figure 8.
This figure illustrates the composition and the mechanism of action of adenine base editing converting A: T to G: C [25].

an intestinal organoid model [20]. CRISPR/Cas9 has also been used to edit *CFTR* in human-induced pluripotent stem cells (iPSCs). This approach provided new models for CF disease, and it helped in the identification of novel drug targets [26].

Added advantages of gene editing over gene therapy are the use of the endogenous cell machinery and the fact that the modifications are permanent for the cell's life time. In addition, the reagents used for one mutation can also be used for any other CF mutation [8].

One of the main concerns when using the CRISPR/Cas9 system is the possibility of off-target effects; therefore, multiple modifications have been made to Cas9 to reduce such effects, e.g., the use of the nickase Cas9-D10A [27] in yeast achieved precise editing with completely undetectable off-target events. Moreover, both the meticulous choice of the target regions and the use of donor DNA templates with asymmetric homology arms have improved the on-target editing [28].

Other obstacles needed to be overcome in order to increase the gene editing efficiency in vivo are similar to those that affect gene transfer vectors such as the delivery mechanism to the stem basal cells of the lungs through the mucus-obstructed CF lung epithelium. Ideally, the target for the gene editing should be the basal airway progenitor cells, but unfortunately, these are "buried" beneath the surface epithelium and it is difficult to reach with the vectors available currently [29]. On the other hand, there is some optimism using different approaches to deliver CRISPR components: either as mRNA or directly as a protein or ribonucleoprotein complexes with modified lentiviral vectors [30].

Another dilemma, unique to CF, is which cells need to be corrected in the airway epithelium to achieve normal lung function and whether the lung stem cells should be targeted. Furthermore, unrestrained high CFTR expression across all the cells of the lung epithelium might have adverse effects, since normally the expression of the CFTR is controlled with tight activation and repression mechanisms [31, 32].

2.3 mRNA-based therapeutics

For CF, the repair of mRNA is a valuable therapeutic technique that was first investigated by Zamecnik et al. [33]. The mRNA repair could be done by either direct repair, exclusion of the defective exon, or a splice site change. The repair of the RNA is done using short double-stranded RNA oligonucleotides, targeting an mRNA sequence between 15 and 40 nucleotides. These oligonucleotides are designed to be specific for every mutation; hence, they might repair or remove the defective RNA [8]. In other studies, the oligonucleotide was designed to target the CFTR splicing mutation 3849 10 kb C-to-T, and it was shown that the defective splicing can be changed to include a cryptic exon and regain the CFTR function [34].

Moreover, ProQR Therapeutics developed QR-010 which targets the F508del mutation. It does not need to cross the nuclear membrane, since it acts in the cytoplasm. QR-010 showed that it can increase the CFTR Cl^- channel activity in homozygous F508del HBE cells. Also, when administered intranasally to mice, it restored the normal potential difference of the lung epithelium [34–37]. QR-010 is currently in a Phase Ib clinical study given as an inhalational drug to treat the homozygous F508del mutation in adults to evaluate its tolerability and its pharmacokinetics [37].

Small interfering RNA (siRNA) is one of the mRNA therapies that is used to silence the epithelial sodium channel, ENaC. It has been shown that upregulation of ENaC in CF leads to dehydration of the airway and formation of thickened mucus [38]. Due to the lack of a proper delivery system, the use of siRNA to transfect epithelial lung CF cells is difficult. However, ENAC silencing by siRNA when formulated with lipid-peptide nanocomplexes was recently reported both in vitro and in vivo [38].

2.4 mRNA therapy

Messenger RNA as a gene therapy approach has several advantages over DNA (as it does not require nuclear localization or transcription) and viruses, since it does not integrate in the genome once inside the cell. For years, scientists have been investigating the possibility of injecting the wild form of the CFTR mRNA to the cytoplasm to act as a template to produce wild-type CFTR protein [9]. Nevertheless, the unstable nature of RNA and its capacity to elicit innate immune responses pose limitations for in vivo applications. However, recent advances in synthetic biology helped alleviate these limitations by modifying the exogenously synthesized mRNAs to mimic their endogenous counterparts. These modifications have led in both an increase in mRNA transfection efficiency, as well as longer protein expression [39].

The immune system has evolved to recognize exogenous RNA, as it can also be found in viruses and other pathogens. Viral single- and double-stranded RNA can induce immune stimulation by interacting with pattern recognition receptors (PRR) tasked with identifying pathogen-associated molecular patterns. Endogenous RNAs evade immune response since they contain modified nucleotides that affect PRR engagement. For example, the incorporation of nucleotide analogs in the RNA sequence, such as 2-thiouridine (2-SU), 5-methylcytidine (5-meC), and 1-methylpseudouridine (m1Ψ), enables them to prevent recognition [40].

Furthermore, to optimize their translational efficiency and stability, the in vitro synthesized mRNAs incorporate a 5′-end modified cap (anti-reverse analogue [modified ARCA]) and a 3′-end poly(A) tail, eventually resembling fully-processed endogenous mRNA molecules [40]. In conclusion, as a result of extensive research, a variety of different chemical modifications of the mRNA in conjunction with its encapsulation into nanoparticles are currently under investigation [41, 42]. A recent study in bronchial epithelial cells has even demonstrated the restoration of chloride secretion using lipid nanoparticles (LNPs) to package and deliver chemically modified CFTR mRNA [43].

3. Drugs for the treatment of cystic fibrosis mutations

There are several drugs that were investigated for the treatment of CF mutations. According to the class of the mutation, different drugs with different mechanisms of action are used. CFTR modulators are small molecule drugs that improve CFTR protein function by a variety of mechanisms [44]. However, those molecules do not treat the main mutation defect of the *CFTR* gene. They can be classified into four categories (**Figure 9**) [45]:

1. The potentiators that increase the gating function and the opening probability of the CFTR Cl^- gates, e.g., Ivacaftor.

2. The correctors that promote protein folding, assisting the transition of the CFTR protein through the cytoplasm to the cell surface, and the rescue of the CFTR protein, e.g., Lumacaftor.

3. The read-through drugs that enable the overriding of the premature termination codons and subsequently lead to complete translation and production of the full length protein, e.g., ataluren.

4. The amplifiers that increase the amount of the CFTR inside the cells and are usually given with other modulators (mentioned above) to increase their efficiency.

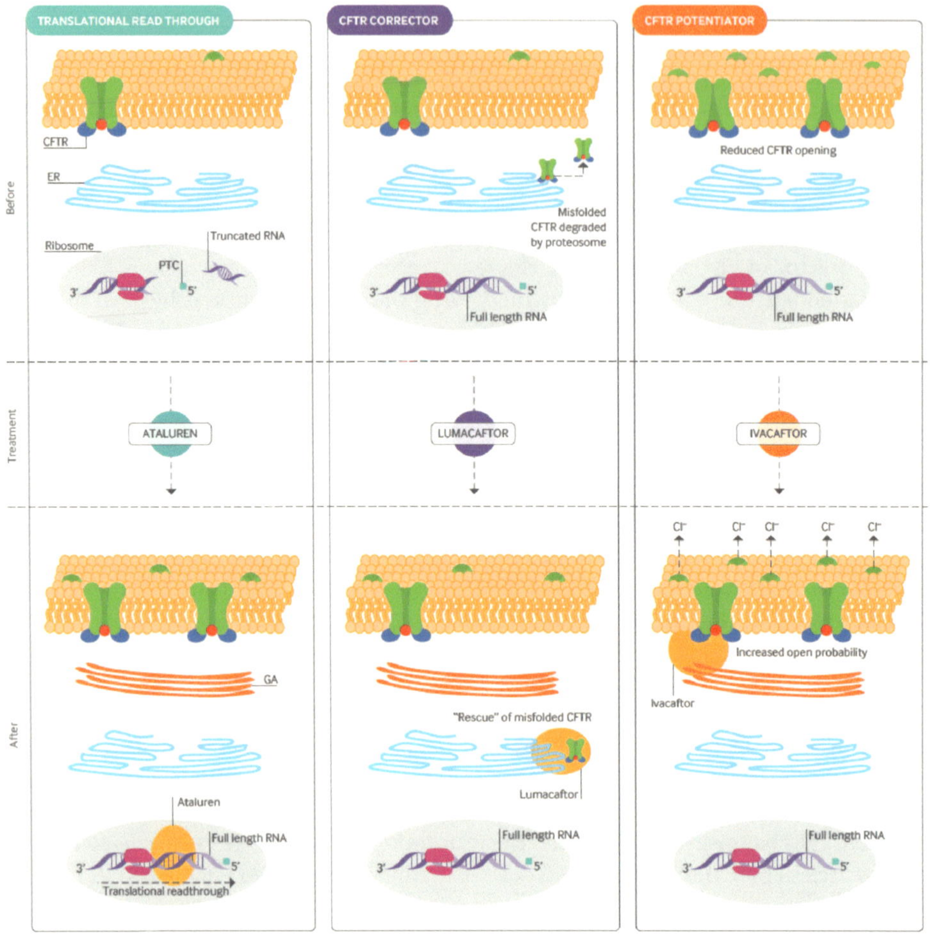

Figure 9.
Different mechanisms of action of drugs that are used to treat the different classes of CF mutations [45]. There is a fourth category of drugs, the amplifiers, which are not depicted here. ER, endoplasmic reticulum; GA, Golgi apparatus; PTC, premature termination codon.

F508del accounts for ~69% of CF-causing alleles [46]. To address this mutation defect, two different forms of drugs are used: CFTR correctors to increase the amount of correctly-folded CFTR protein and CFTR potentiators that improve the gating mechanism of the apical CFTR protein [47]. When combined together, they restore the Cl^- transport and improve the airway mucociliary clearance [48]. The commercially available formulations of these two drugs are the corrector Lumacaftor (VX-809) and the potentiator Ivacaftor (VX-770). When administered alone in patients homozygous for F508del, Lumacaftor lead to a modest, yet statistically significant reduction of ≥10 mmol/L in the sweat chloride concentration, but no other improvements in lung function (FEV_1) and quality of life (CFQ-R) were observed [49]. On the other hand, in patients with the G551D mutation, Ivacaftor lead to an all-around improvement. In detail, after 48 weeks, the treated patients demonstrated an overall increase in BMI and quality of life markers, a 10.6% increase in FEV_1, as well as a decrease of 48.1 mmol/L in sweat chloride levels, making Ivacaftor the first agent to achieve a reduction to values below the diagnostic threshold for CF (60 mmol/L). As a result, Ivacaftor was approved for the treatment of the Class III CF mutations in 2012 [50, 51]. The combination of both, which is called Orkambi, is currently available for CF patients as it proved beneficial for homozygous F508del mutation treatment. To elaborate, in addition to a significant general improvement in the clinical picture of the disease, such as increased BMI and CFQ-R, and a decreased rate of exacerbations, a 5% improvement of FEV_1, when compared to the placebo, was observed [52, 53]. In 2019, a triple combination therapy consisting of the correctors Elexacaftor and Tezacaftor and the potentiator Ivacaftor (called Trikafta and developed by Vertex Pharmaceuticals) was tested in a double blind, randomized phase 3 clinical trial, demonstrating remarkable results. Among others, a significant increase in CFQ-R and a favorable safety profile. Moreover, there was a 10.4% increase in FEV_1 and a considerable improvement in sweat chloride concentration, with a mean decrease of 43.4 mmol/L, achieving values below the diagnostic threshold for CF. Subsequently, Trikafta was approved by the FDA as a treatment among patients aged 12 years or older with the F508del mutation [53].

Furthermore, a number of proteins based on proteostasis modulation have been identified as useful drug targets for CF therapy [54–56]. Hsp90 and AHA1 are thought to have a role in CFTR folding and degradation. It was found that treatment with Hsp90-AHA1 inhibitors combined with Lumacaftor was more effective than Lumacaftor alone [56].

Ataluren is another drug that was used to facilitate the read-through of nonsense mutations in Duchene Muscular Dystrophy. However, a randomized clinical phase II trial showed no significant efficacy of Ataluren in the treatment of CF [57]. ELX-02 is another drug that is recently developed by ELoxx Pharmaceuticals for its read-through effects. It is currently in a phase 2 clinical trial involving CF patients [58].

Another possible drug target is endoplasmic reticulum-associated degradation (ERAD), including chaperone proteins and ubiquitin complexes. RNF5 (also known as RMA1) was found to be important in the protein folding and NBD domain synthesis [59].

Interestingly, due to the presence of more than 2000 mutations in *CFTR*, the use of "theratyping" for the patient becomes of value. The term "theratype" is described as classifying the CFTR variants according to their response to the corrector and potentiator drugs. More recently, this term is used to classify the mutations according to their characterization and their response to CFTR modulators across many model systems, which include functional and biochemical characterization [45]. Theratyping is also used to predict the clinical outcome of the patient toward the drug by the in vitro studies [45].

4. Nonviral delivery vectors

For a long time, viral vectors dominated the fields of gene therapy and vector development, mainly due to their very high efficiency. However, over the last years, novel approaches in vector design and recent advances in microfluidics have turned nonviral vectors into a promising method of drug and gene delivery [60, 61]. There are multiple materials that can be used to create nonviral vectors, including liposomes, which allow the delivery of the nucleic acids inside the lung epithelial cells. Liposomes are spherical vesicles composed of two layers of phospholipids with a hydrophilic core. They are normally formulated with natural lipids and possess no immunogenicity [62].

Nonviral vectors have the advantages of simple large-scale production and a large capacity for nucleic acids as cargos. Furthermore, low host immunogenicity and the ability to maintain their efficiency even after repeated administration render them a popular alternative to their viral counterparts. In addition, recent advances in vector technology have yielded molecules and techniques with even higher transfection efficiencies [60, 61]. These new vectors can be used to deliver small molecules such as siRNAs, miRNAs, or even small therapeutic molecules and drugs, as well as bigger molecules like mRNA, minicircle, and plasmid DNA.

The cationic lipid-based vectors are an effective delivery approach for the CRISPR/Cas9 system but only after local administration [62]. However, the main problem about liposomes as drug delivery vectors for the treatment of CF or any chronic obstructive disease remains the development of inhalational formulations which can be delivered by nebulization. The nebulizer can alter the stability of the liposomes and cause their aggregation [63]. Therefore, several methods have been developed to stabilize the liposomal formulations such as lyophilisation [64] or use of dry powder inhaler (DPI) liposomal formulations which have shown promising results for drug administration in the lung, but those are still in an early development stage [65]. Targeted liposome-peptide nanocomplexes have been successfully nebulized, offering another alternative [66, 67].

Additionally, mucus-penetrating nanoparticles have emerged as a suitable vector to deliver various drugs and nucleic acids across the thick mucus barrier in cystic fibrosis. In CF, targeted mucus-penetrating nanocomplexes successfully delivered siRNA against ENAC in the airway epithelium and decreased the Na^+ reabsorption, thus restoring the clearance of the mucus and regaining the function of cilia [38, 68]. Mucus-penetrating NPs have a small size which leads to a lower mucus surface tension and easy penetrance. Also, they are coated with polyethylene glycol (PEG) which is electrically neutral and lead to an enhancement of the penetrance of the thick mucus of CF [69]. PEGylated nanoparticles loaded with Ivacaftor were formulated to test the drug uptake capacity of CF artificial mucus (CF-AM) on human bronchial epithelial (16-HBE) cells [70]. It was found that there was a higher release and uptake of Ivacaftor by 12% compared to Ivacaftor alone. In light of these results, the PEGylated mucus-penetrating NPs are considered a good vehicle to deliver the CFTR modulators through pulmonary administration to treat CF patients [70]. However, in order to be effective, the size of mucus-penetrating NPs should be small enough to penetrate mucus and big enough to prevent rapid exhalation and expulsion from the lung. Moreover, in order to increase their efficacy, certain parameters must be considered such as the nanoparticle morphology and their surface properties [71].

In summary, both viral and nonviral vectors are used to introduce different nucleic acids into the cell. Though the design of viral vectors has improved in the last few years and they have become more efficient, the immunogenicity and safety concerns still remain a big issue. On the other hand, the nonviral vectors offer safe and low-cost therapies with increased transfection efficiencies. Further improvements and optimization of these therapies and delivery vehicles could lead to a great outcome for CF [72].

5. CF animal models, organoids and iPSCs

Having an animal model is a crucial step to understand the disease pathogenesis, progression, and to test new drugs. The CFTR-knockout pigs and ferrets were generated approximately 15 years ago [73]. These species have a similar lung biology to humans because their submucosal glands are in their cartilaginous parts of the lung. On the contrary, rats and mice have their submucosal glands in the trachea, and rabbits do not have glands at all [74].

Among other in vitro cell culture models, one that has particular value in CF is the use of organoids, which have become a very useful model for CF research [75]. Organoids are 3D cultures of the lung progenitor cells grown in the presence of appropriate medium. They grow also with supporting cells that organize in a very similar way as the in vivo organs. In CF research, organoids of the intestinal and respiratory systems are currently used to screen and test the newest drugs for CF [20]. Moreover, the intestinal organoids have been used as a model for the CRISPR/Cas9 technique [20].

These models could also be used potentially for testing gene editing-based therapeutics in CF [8, 76]. Another therapeutic option is to directly edit the progenitor cells in the lung epithelium in vivo, but a CRISPR editing system in CF lung in vivo has yet to be reported [8].

Human embryonic stem cells (ESCs) and iPSCs are newer models that can be used in CF. iPSCs are obtained by somatic cell reprogramming and differentiating these cells into specific human tissues [77]. The iPSCs can produce cell lines with the different rare CF mutations. The CRISPR/Cas9 technique was efficiently used to correct the CFTR F508del in patient-derived iPSCs that were differentiated to proximal airway cells [78].

6. Conclusion

Cystic fibrosis is a good example of how a deeper understanding of the genetics of disease can lead to personalized therapy for each patient. Continued efforts to develop better viral and nanoparticle-based nonviral vectors and produce novel gene editing with CRISPR/Cas9 are always investigated. Along with the advancement in the production of CF animal and in vitro human models and the presence of different electrophysiological methods such as transepithelial potential difference (TPD), all these give the promise and hope for the future of CF patients. Certainly, the recent use of organoids will be essential to personalized genetic medicine. This chapter has presented the past and current research that shows that the concept of genetic medicine can become a reality for CF patients in the near future.

Author details

Salsabil Elboraie, Konstantinos N. Kafetzis, Rajeev Shrivastava and Aristides D. Tagalakis*
Department of Biology, Edge Hill University, Ormskirk, UK

*Address all correspondence to: aristides.tagalakis@edgehill.ac.uk

References

[1] Wang Y et al. Understanding how cystic fibrosis mutations disrupt CFTR function: From single molecules to animal models. The International Journal of Biochemistry & Cell Biology. 2014;**52**(1):47-57

[2] Sheppard DN, Welsh MJ. Structure and function of the CFTR chloride channel. Physiological Reviews. 1999;**79**(1 Suppl):23

[3] Vallières E et al. Cystic fibrosis gene mutations: Evaluation and assessment of disease severity. Advances in Genomics and Genetics. 2014;**4**(1):161-172

[4] Brodlie M et al. Targeted therapies to improve CFTR function in cystic fibrosis. Genome Medicine. 2015;**7**(14):101

[5] De Boeck K et al. Progress in therapies for cystic fibrosis. The Lancet Respiratory Medicine. 2016;**4**(8):662-674

[6] Fanen P et al. Genetics of cystic fibrosis: CFTR mutation classifications toward genotype-based CF therapies. The International Journal of Biochemistry & Cell Biology. 2014;**52**:94-102

[7] Amaral MD et al. Progress in therapies for cystic fibrosis. The Lancet Respiratory Medicine. 2016;**4**(8):662-674

[8] Alton EW et al. Genetic medicines for CF: Hype versus reality. Pediatric Pulmonology. 2016;**51**(S44):S5-S17

[9] Griesenbach U, U.K.C.F.G.T. Consortium, et al. Gene transfer to the lung: Lessons learned from more than 2 decades of CF gene therapy. Advanced Drug Delivery Reviews. 2009;**61**(2):128-139

[10] Griesenbach U et al. Cystic fibrosis gene therapy in the UK and elsewhere. Human Gene Therapy. 2015;**26**(5):266-275

[11] Alton E et al. Repeated nebulisation of non-viral CFTR gene therapy in patients with cystic fibrosis: A randomised, double-blind, placebo-controlled, phase 2b trial. The Lancet Respiratory Medicine. 2015;**3**(9):684-691

[12] Kobayashi M et al. Reversion in vivo after inoculation of a molecular proviral DNA clone of simian immunodeficiency virus with a cytotoxic-T-lymphocyte escape mutation. Journal of Virology. 2005;**79**(17):11529-11532

[13] Alton EW et al. Preparation for a first-in-man lentivirus trial in patients with cystic fibrosis. Thorax. 2017;**72**(2):137-147

[14] Yan Z et al. A novel chimeric adenoassociated virus 2/human bocavirus 1 parvovirus vector efficiently transduces human airway epithelia. Molecular Therapy. 2013;**21**(12):2181-2194

[15] Hsu PD et al. Development and applications of CRISPR-Cas9 for genome engineering. Cell. 2014;**157**(6):1262-1278

[16] Gaj T et al. C.F., ZFN, TALEN, and CRISPR/Cas-based methods for genome engineering. Trends in Biotechnology. 2013;**31**(7):397-405

[17] Loureiro A et al. CRISPR-Cas: Converting a bacterial defence mechanism into a state-of-the-art genetic manipulation tool. Antibiotics (Basel, Switzerland). 2019;**8**(1):18-25

[18] Ott de Bruin L et al. Rapid generation of novel models of RAG1 deficiency by CRISPR/Cas9-induced mutagenesis in murine zygotes. Oncotarget. 2016;**7**(11):12962-12974

[19] Redman M et al. What is CRISPR/Cas9? Archives of disease in childhood.

ADC Education and Practice Edition. 2016;**101**(4):213-215

[20] Schwank G et al. Functional repair of CFTR by CRISPR/Cas9 in intestinal stem cell organoids of cystic fibrosis patients. Cell Stem Cell. 2013;**13**(6):653-658

[21] Eid A et al. CRISPR base editors: Genome editing without double-stranded breaks. The Biochemical Journal. 2018;**475**(11):1955-1964

[22] Gearing M. Single base editing with CRISPR. Addgene Blog. 2016. Available from: https://blog.addgene.org/single-base-editing-with-crispr [Accessed: 18 May 2020]

[23] Mention K et al. Gene and base editing as a therapeutic option for cystic fibrosis—Learning from other diseases. Genes (Basel). 2019;**10**(5):E387

[24] Gaudelli NM et al. Programmable base editing of A*T to G*C in genomic DNA without DNA cleavage. Nature. 2017;**551**(7681):464-471

[25] Gearing M. CRISPR 101: RNA editing with Cas13 and repair. Addgene Blog. 2017. Available from: https://blog.addgene.org/crispr-101-rna-editing-with-cas13-and-repair [Accessed: 18 May 2020]

[26] Firth AL et al. Functional gene correction for cystic fibrosis in lung epithelial cells generated from patient iPSCs. Cell Reports. 2015;**12**(9):1385-1390

[27] Satomura A et al. Precise genome-wide base editing by the CRISPR Nickase system in yeast. Scientific Reports. 2017;**7**(1):2095

[28] Miyaoka Y et al. Systematic quantification of HDR and NHEJ reveals effects of locus, nuclease, and cell type on genome-editing. Scientific Reports. 2016;**6**(1):23549

[29] Munye MM et al. Minicircle DNA provides enhanced and prolonged transgene expression following airway gene transfer. Scientific Reports. 2016;**6**(1):23125

[30] Choi JG et al. Lentivirus pre-packed with Cas9 protein for safer gene editing. Gene Therapy. 2016;**23**(7):627-633

[31] Zhang Z, Leir SH, Harris A. Immune mediators regulate CFTR expression through a bifunctional airway-selective enhancer. Molecular and Cellular Biology. 2013;**33**(15):2843-2853

[32] Zhang Z et al. Oxidative stress regulates CFTR gene expression in human airway epithelial cells through a distal antioxidant response element. American Journal of Respiratory Cell and Molecular Biology. 2015;**52**(3):387-396

[33] Zamecnik PC et al. Reversal of cystic fibrosis phenotype in a cultured Delta508 cystic fibrosis transmembrane conductance regulator cell line by oligonucleotide insertion. Proceedings of the National Academy of Sciences of the United States of America. 2004;**101**(21):8150-8155

[34] Nissim-Rafinia M et al. Cellular and viral splicing factors can modify the splicing pattern of CFTR transcripts carrying splicing mutations. Human Molecular Genetics. 2000;**9**(12):1771-1778

[35] Swildens J et al. QR-010, an antisense oligonuleotide, restores CFTR function in delta F508 cell cultures. Pediatric Pulmonology. 2014;**49**:301-302

[36] Beumer W et al. Qr-010 restores Cftr-mediated chloride transport in F508del Cf mice assessed by transepithelial nasal potential difference. Pediatric Pulmonology. 2014;**49**:227-228

[37] Henig N et al. Qr-010, an Rna therapy, restores Cftr function in the saliva secretion assay. American Journal of Respiratory and Critical Care Medicine. 2015;**191**(14):100-106

[38] Manunta MDI et al. Delivery of ENaC siRNA to epithelial cells mediated by a targeted nanocomplex: A therapeutic strategy for cystic fibrosis. Scientific Reports. 2017;**7**(1):700

[39] Boucher RC. Cystic fibrosis: A disease of vulnerability to airway surface dehydration. Trends in Molecular Medicine. 2007;**13**(6):231-240

[40] Sahin U et al. mRNA-based therapeutics—Developing a new class of drugs. Nature Reviews. Drug Discovery. 2014;**13**(10):759-780

[41] Mahiny AJ et al. In vivo genome editing using nuclease-encoding mRNA corrects SP-B deficiency. Nature Biotechnology. 2015;**33**(6):584-586

[42] Mays LE et al. Modified Foxp3 mRNA protects against asthma through an IL-10-dependent mechanism. The Journal of Clinical Investigation. 2013;**123**(3):1216-1228

[43] Robinson E et al. Lipid nanoparticle-delivered chemically modified mRNA restores chloride secretion in cystic fibrosis. Molecular Therapy. 2018;**26**(8):2034-2046

[44] Clancy JP et al. CFTR modulator theratyping: Current status, gaps and future directions. Journal of Cystic Fibrosis. 2019;**18**(1):22-34

[45] Quon BS et al. New and emerging targeted therapies for cystic fibrosis. BMJ. 2016;**352**:i859

[46] Castellani C et al. Consensus on the use and interpretation of cystic fibrosis mutation analysis in clinical practice. Journal of Cystic Fibrosis. 2008;**7**(3):179-196

[47] Lukacs GL et al. CFTR: Folding, misfolding and correcting the DeltaF508 conformational defect. Trends in Molecular Medicine. 2012;**18**(2):81-91

[48] Li H et al. Therapeutic approaches to CFTR dysfunction: From discovery to drug development. Journal of Cystic Fibrosis. 2018;**17**(2S):S14-S21

[49] Clancy JP et al. Results of a phase IIa study of VX-809, an investigational CFTR corrector compound, in subjects with cystic fibrosis homozygous for the F508del-CFTR mutation. Thorax. 2012;**67**(1):12-18

[50] Ramsey BW et al. A CFTR potentiator in patients with cystic fibrosis and the G551D mutation. The New England Journal of Medicine. 2011;**365**(18):1663-1672

[51] Wainwright CE et al. Lumacaftor-ivacaftor in patients with cystic fibrosis homozygous for Phe508del CFTR. The New England Journal of Medicine. 2015;**373**(18):1783-1784

[52] Boyle MP et al. A CFTR corrector (lumacaftor) and a CFTR potentiator (ivacaftor) for treatment of patients with cystic fibrosis who have a phe508del CFTR mutation: A phase 2 randomised controlled trial. The Lancet Respiratory Medicine. 2014;**2**(7):527-538

[53] Heijerman HGM et al. Efficacy and safety of the elexacaftor plus tezacaftor plus ivacaftor combination regimen in people with cystic fibrosis homozygous for the F508del mutation: A double-blind, randomised, phase 3 trial. Lancet. 2019;**394**(10212):1940-1948

[54] Balch WE et al. Adapting proteostasis for disease intervention. Science. 2008;**319**(5865):916-919

[55] Sondo E et al. RNF5, DAB2 and friends: Novel drug targets for cystic fibrosis. Current Pharmaceutical Design. 2017;**23**(1):176-186

[56] Ihrig V et al. Identifying inhibitors of the Hsp90-Aha1 protein complex, a potential target to drug cystic fibrosis, by alpha technology. SLAS Discovery. 2017;**22**(7):923-928

[57] Zainal Abidin N et al. Ataluren in cystic fibrosis: Development, clinical studies and where are we now? Expert Opinion on Pharmacotherapy. 2017;**18**(13).1363-1371

[58] Leubitz A et al. Safety, tolerability, and pharmacokinetics of single ascending doses of ELX-02, a potential treatment for genetic disorders caused by nonsense mutations, in healthy volunteers. Clinical Pharmacology in Drug Development. 2019;**8**(8):984-994

[59] Younger JM et al. Sequential quality-control checkpoints triage misfolded cystic fibrosis transmembrane conductance regulator. Cell. 2006;**126**(3):571-582

[60] Ramamoorth M, Narvekar A. Non-viral vectors in gene therapy—An overview. Journal of Clinical and Diagnostic Research. 2015;**9**(1):GE01-GE06

[61] Alavi SE et al. Drug delivery of hydroxyurea to breast cancer using liposomes. Indian Journal of Clinical Biochemistry. 2013;**28**(3):299-302

[62] Li L et al. Non-viral delivery systems for CRISPR/Cas9-based genome editing: Challenges and opportunities. Biomaterials. 2018;**171**:207-218

[63] d'Angelo I et al. Improving the efficacy of inhaled drugs in cystic fibrosis: Challenges and emerging drug delivery strategies. Advanced Drug Delivery Reviews. 2014;**75**:92-111

[64] Chen C et al. An overview of liposome lyophilization and its future potential. Journal of Controlled Release. 2010;**142**(3):299-311

[65] Velino C et al. Nanomedicine approaches for the pulmonary treatment of cystic fibrosis. Frontiers in Bioengineering and Biotechnology. 2019;**7**:406-410

[66] Manunta MD et al. Airway deposition of nebulized gene delivery nanocomplexes monitored by radioimaging agents. American Journal of Respiratory Cell and Molecular Biology. 2013;**49**(3):471-480

[67] Manunta MD et al. Nebulisation of receptor-targeted nanocomplexes for gene delivery to the airway epithelium. PLoS One. 2011;**6**(10):e26768

[68] Tagalakis AD et al. Effective silencing of ENaC by siRNA delivered with epithelial-targeted nanocomplexes in human cystic fibrosis cells and in mouse lung. Thorax. 2018;**73**(9):847-856

[69] Ong V et al. Nanomedicine for cystic fibrosis. SLAS Technology. 2019;**24**(2):169-180

[70] Porsio B et al. Mucus and cell-penetrating nanoparticles embedded in nano-into-micro formulations for pulmonary delivery of ivacaftor in patients with cystic fibrosis. ACS Applied Materials & Interfaces. 2018;**10**(1):165-181

[71] Paranjpe M et al. Nanoparticle-mediated pulmonary drug delivery: A review. International Journal of Molecular Sciences. 2014;**15**(4):5852-5873

[72] Gomes Dos Reis L et al. Inhaled gene delivery: A formulation and delivery approach. Expert Opinion on Drug Delivery. 2017;**14**(3):319-330

[73] Rogers CS et al. Production of CFTR-null and CFTR-Delta F508 heterozygous pigs by adeno-associated virus-mediated gene targeting and somatic cell nuclear transfer. The

Journal of Clinical Investigation. 2008;**118**(4):1571-1577

[74] Rogers CS et al. Disruption of the CFTR gene produces a model of cystic fibrosis in newborn pigs. Science. 2008;**321**(5897):1837-1841

[75] Rosen BH et al. Animal and model systems for studying cystic fibrosis. Journal of Cystic Fibrosis. 2018;**17**(2):S28-S34

[76] Butler CR et al. Rapid expansion of human epithelial stem cells suitable for airway tissue engineering. American Journal of Respiratory and Critical Care Medicine. 2016;**194**(2):156-168

[77] Martin U. Pluripotent stem cells for disease modeling and drug screening: New perspectives for treatment of cystic fibrosis. Molecular and Cellular Pediatrics. 2015;**2**(1):15

[78] Firth AL et al. Functional gene correction for cystic fibrosis in lung epithelial cells generated from patient iPSCs. Cell Reports. 2015;**12**(9):1385-1390